GLUTEN FREE COOKBOOK

Delicious and Simple Dishes From the Large Recipe and Baking World

(The Ultimate Guide to Gluten-free Cookbook)

Cameron Herrera

Published by Sharon Lohan

© Cameron Herrera

All Rights Reserved

Gluten Free Cookbook: Delicious and Simple Dishes From the Large Recipe and Baking World (The Ultimate Guide to Gluten-free Cookbook)

ISBN 978-1-990334-12-2

All rights reserved. No part of this guide may be reproduced in any form without permission in writing from the publisher except in the case of brief quotations embodied in critical articles or reviews.

Legal & Disclaimer

The information contained in this book is not designed to replace or take the place of any form of medicine or professional medical advice. The information in this book has been provided for educational and entertainment purposes only.

The information contained in this book has been compiled from sources deemed reliable, and it is accurate to the best of the Author's knowledge; however, the Author cannot guarantee its accuracy and validity and cannot be held liable for any errors or omissions. Changes are periodically made to this book. You must consult your doctor or get professional medical advice before using any of the suggested remedies, techniques, or information in this book.

Table of contents

Part 1 1
Introduction 2
Chapter 1: What is Gluten? 3
Chapter 2: Gluten Myths Debunked 5
Chapter 3: How a Gluten-Free Diet can Help Promote Weight-Loss 7
Chapter 4: Gluten-Intolerance: One Cause, Many Diseases 10
Chapter 5: What is Coeliac Disease? 15
Chapter 6: Why Gluten-Free Flours are Better than Commonly Used Wheat Flour! 17
Chapter 7: GF Dining - Tips for Dining Out while on a Gluten-Free Diet 22
Chapter 8: 8 Tips to Make your Gluten-Free Lifestyle Much Easier 26
Chapter 9: Kids on a Gluten-Free Diet: Tips to Make Life Easier 29
GLUTEN-FREE SCHOOL LUNCH IDEAS FOR THE KIDDOS 29
KID FRIENDLY GLUTEN-FREE SNACKS 32
Homemade Potato Chips & Ranch Dip 34
Chapter 10: Benefits of a Gluten-Free Diet in Children with Autism 36

Chapter 11: Gluten Intolerance VS Lactose Intolerance 37

Chapter 12: Can Coeliac Disease Affect the Brain? 40

Chapter 13: The story of Jess Madden: a Doctor and Coeliac Patient 43

Chapter 14: Your Guide to a Gluten-Free Meal Plan .. 48

Chapter 15: Gluten-Free on a Budget 52

Chapter 16: Incredibly Healthy Gluten Free Super-Foods 54

Chapter 17: Delicious Gluten-Free Recipes (Desserts Included!) 66

Gluten-Free Recipes 66

G-Free Banana Pancakes 66

Easy and Delicious Breakfast Quinoa 68

Deliciously Fluffy Gluten-free Pancakes (makes 10 servings) 69

Breakfast Sausage 70

Blueberry Oatmeal Breakfast-smoothie 71

Protein Packed Cherry-Quinoa Bars 71

Spanish Breakfast Tortilla 74

Vegetable and Egg Scramble with Fontina Cheese 75

Avocado and Egg Breakfast Burrito 76

The Perfect Lunch Salad 77

Grill Marinated Shrimp 79

Stuffed Peppers	80
Bacon-wrapped Pork Roast Recipe	82
Sirloin Steak with Garlic Butter	83
Baked Kale Chips (make a great addition to any lunch!)	84
Caramel Apple Pork Chops	85
Black Beans and Quinoa	86
Italian Style Fish Fillets	88
Juicy Seasoned Roasted Chicken	89
Shrimp and Cheddar Grits	90
Baked Shrimp in Tomato Feta Sauce Recipe	91
Brown Butter Harvest Cake with Vanilla Nut Cream	92
Raspberry Lemon Cheesecake Bites	96
Gluten-Free Garbanzo Bean Chocolate Cake	97
Gluten-Free Chocolate Chip Cookies	99
Strawberry Soup	100
Chocolate Pudding Cups	100
Peach and Raspberry Parfait	101
Conclusion	103
Part 2	104
Introduction	105
Chapter 1: Gluten free Breads	108
Almond Buns	108
Garlic Dill Dinner Rolls	109

French bread (baguette) 110
Sandwich Bread 112
Zucchini Bread 113
Chapter 2: Gluten free Dips Recipes...................... 115
Roasted Sweet Onion Dip 115
Hummus 116
Healthy Broccoli Guacamole: 117
Tomato salsa 117
Creamy Curry Cashew Dip..................................... 118
Baba Ghanoush... 118
Chapter 3: Gluten free Smoothie Recipes 121
Apple Pie Green Smoothie: 121
Cranberry & raspberry smoothie 121
Mango, Lime n Jalapeno Smoothie: 123
Energy Boosting Smoothie 124
Flat - Belly Smoothie 124
Blueberry Tofu Protein Smoothie: 125
Chapter 4: Gluten free Breakfast Recipes 126
All in one Baked Mushrooms 126
Smoked Salmon Frittata:....................................... 127
Rice and Raisin Breakfast Pudding: 128
Quinoa Porridge:... 129
Potato & Paprika Tortilla....................................... 130

Chickpea Pancakes: 132
Chapter 5: Gluten free Salad Recipes 133
The Big Salad: 133
Edamame Salad: 135
Grapefruit, Agave & Pistachio salad 136
Spicy Slaw 137
Chapter 6: Gluten free Snacks Recipes 138
Cauliflower Tostadas: 138
Zucchini Pizza bites: 139
Puffed Quinoa Peanut Butter Balls: 140
Chapter 7: Gluten free Appetizers' Recipes 141
Spiced Sweet Potato Wedges 141
Bruschetta with Warm Tomatoes 143
Beef Teriyaki Crisps with Wasabi Mayonnaise 145
Marinated Shrimp on the Grill 147
Lemon-Caper Parmesan Potato Salad Bites 148
Chapter 8: Gluten free Soups Recipes 150
Moroccan Lentil Soup: 150
Pesto Chicken Soup: 152
Cream of Mushroom Soup: 153
Turkey Tortilla Soup 154
Gazpacho 156
Chapter 9: Gluten free Main Course 157

Authentic Spanish Paella 157

Takikomi Gohan (Japanese Mixed Rice): 159

Tandoori Chicken: 161

Chicken and Broccoli 162

Shallow Poached Trout: 164

Smoked haddock with lemon & dill lentils 165

Persian lamb Tagine 167

Apple Cinnamon Pork Chops 170

Beef Ragu: 172

Teriyaki Tofu and Mushrooms 173

Chickpea Bajane 175

Soft Tacos with Green Chile–Cilantro Rice and Egg .. 177

Chapter 10: Gluten free Side Dishes 179

Zucchini Pasta 179

Zoodles (Zucchini noodles) 180

Bacon and Cheddar Mashed Potatoes 181

Balsamic Roasted Asparagus 183

Mexican Quinoa 184

Braised Kale with Bacon and Cider 185

Chapter 11: Gluten free Desserts Recipes 186

Chocolate Pudding: 186

Conclusion 188

Part 1

Introduction

This book contains proven steps and strategies on how to improve the quality of your health and overall well-being through benefitting from the many favorable advantages of a gluten-free diet.

This book is your ultimate guide to a gluten-free lifestyle, and will provide you with a plethora of useful and valuable information about the amazing benefits of going gluten-free. This includes sharing the positive impacts it has towards a number of digestive issues and discomforts, weight-loss and even complex conditions like Autism. It will provide you with many useful tips and support, (including a list of delicious and flavorful gluten-free recipes!) while informing you about everything you need to know about the decision to maintain a gluten-free lifestyle.

Thanks again for downloading this book, I hope you enjoy it!

Chapter 1: What is Gluten?

A gluten free diet has become a popular addition to the world of various new age, trendy diets. However, making a conscious decision to stick to a gluten free diet is far more beneficial (and in some cases, absolutely crucial) to your health than a ridiculous diet fad like the "baby food diet", which is nothing more than an unreasonable waste of time.

WHAT IS GLUTEN?

Gluten is a protein most commonly found in wheat, barley and rye, and is found in a wide array of foods such as breads, baked goods, soups, pasta, cereals, salad dressings, sauces, roux, beer, malt and food dyes. It is the substance responsible for the elastic texture of dough, and acts like glue by holding food together and maintaining its shape. Gluten is found in a large portion of foods - even in the foods you'd least expect.

The term "gluten" refers to wheat endosperm, which is a type of tissue produced in seeds that is ground to make flour. Gluten is known to provide foods with an elastic, chewy consistency.

Gluten is actually composed of two different proteins, although it is typically referred to as a single protein. Gluten is composed of gliadin (a prolamin protein) and glutenin (a glutelin protein). Although gluten is sometimes thought to be specifically linked to wheat, it is also found in other grains like barley and rye, since these grains also contain protein composites made from promalins and glutelins.

A gluten-free diet eliminates all sources of gluten, and all foods that contain protein composites made from promalins and glutelins, including bread, pasta, rolls and oat-based foods.

Chapter 2: Gluten Myths Debunked

As with anything, there are many myths about gluten that cause a number of misconceptions about the substance. Here is a list of common myths and misconceptions about gluten.

Going gluten-free means saying goodbye to flavor, and having to eat bland, tasteless foods.

This is definitely one of the biggest misconceptions about a gluten-free diet. Just because going gluten-free requires saying goodbye to foods like wheat bread and pasta doesn't by any means indicate that you are doomed to eat bland, boring foods for the rest of your life. For instance, fresh or dried herbs and spices certainly add plenty of flavor to meals and are a perfectly acceptable staple in a gluten-free diet. Does a deliciously seasoned meal of grilled chicken with a side of buttery, creamy mashed potatoes and flavorful sautéed vegetables sound "bland and tasteless" to you? Didn't think so!

Eating gluten causes cancer.

Unless you suffer from coeliacs disease, or have an abnormal immune system response whenever you consume gluten, it is very unlikely that you will develop cancer - or any other serious illness as a result of eating gluten. People with a coeliacs disease - a serious condition involving severe gluten-intolerance - could very well have a risk of developing an illness because of the fact that their bodies simply cannot handle the substance to the point where it damages their small intestine and prevents them from properly absorbing vital nutrients from their food that are necessary for overall health and well-being. However, if your immune system doesn't have an abnormally sensitive response to gluten, consuming it will not pose as a dangerous red flag to your health.

Coeliac disease and gluten sensitivity are the same thing.

This is absolutely untrue! Coeliac disease is an autoimmune disorder in which the body produces antibodies and attacks the small intestines whenever gluten is consumed. This does not at all occur in those with only a mere sensitivity to gluten, nor is it a precursor to coeliacs disease or a mild form of it.

There are many myths about gluten, and it's important to be aware of the medically-proven, true facts about gluten, especially if it's necessary for you to maintain a gluten-free lifestyle.

Chapter 3: How a Gluten-Free Diet can Help Promote Weight-Loss

Making the decision to stick to a gluten-free diet can actually help you lose weight, regardless of whether or not you're gluten-intolerant! This is mainly because you're eliminating the fattening starch-laden foods that are making it increasingly difficult for you to trim off those extra few pounds. Gluten is loaded in almost every "bad for you" food. These offenders include morning favorites like doughnuts, bagels, muffins and pastries, as well as greasy late-night cravings like pizza and burgers. A gluten-free diet eliminates all of these weight-gain instigators and replaces them with healthy, waistline-friendly substitutes consisting of lean proteins, healthy fats and plenty of nutrient-packed fruits and vegetables.

In many cases, people who switch to a gluten-free diet also find themselves effortlessly shedding 15-20 pounds (over 1 stone/5-6 kilograms) in only a month, simply by eliminating one of the most common sources of gluten: wheat!

Many experts - notably cardiologist Dr. William Davis, author of "Wheat Belly" argue that wheat (and not just the gluten found in wheat) actually increases your appetite, which leads to weight-gain. Dr. Davis has explained that wheat contains appetite-stimulating compounds which encourage your body to produce more insulin, a hormone that can cause the body to store fat. Eliminating gluten is known to decrease your body's levels of insulin production, which in turn reduces appetite and curbs intense cravings. The result? Significantly improved weight-loss results.

However, while gluten-free eating habits can definitely boost weight-loss, it's important to avoid overeating and stick to a regime of well-balanced, reduced calorie meals to achieve maximum weight-loss results while on a gluten-free diet. Here is an included example of a gluten-free, 1,500 calorie daily meal plan, which can cause you to lose up to 4 pounds a week! You may need more or less calories, depending on your age, gender, height, and level of exercise. There are free sites like Calorie Counter that provide you with an estimated amount of calories you need per day to lose weight, depending on your body type and activity levels.

1,500-calorie meal plan:

Breakfast:

Omelet - made with two eggs and two egg whites and filled with 1/2 cup sautéed onions, bell peppers and mushrooms.

1 cup of honey dew melon

1 slice of gluten-free toast topped with 1/4 of an avocado and salt and pepper to taste

Morning Snack:

1 ounce of almonds (or any nuts of your choice) and 4 ounces of baby carrots

Lunch:

3 ounces of skinless, grilled chicken breast

1 cup of tossed salad with 1 tablespoon of vinegar and oil salad dressing

1 cup of skim milk

Afternoon Snack:

1 medium nectarine or 1/2 cup of fresh berries

Dinner:

5 ounce sole, baked, with fresh lemon

1 cup of quinoa

1 cup of steamed broccoli with one teaspoon of minced garlic, and one tablespoon of chopped walnuts or slivered almonds

A gluten-free diet alone will not act as a magical key to weight-loss, but it will certainly aid you in shedding extra weight, as it will prevent excess cravings and will eliminate a large group of fattening, calorie-laden diet offenders that make it especially challenging for you to reach your ideal weight. A gluten-free diet accompanied by well-balanced, calorie conscious meal choices will definitely provide you with exceptionally powerful, effective weight-loss results, while contributing to an overall healthier, happier you.

Chapter 4: Gluten-Intolerance: One Cause, Many Diseases

For many individuals, the benefits of a gluten-free lifestyle generally translate to improved health, as well as increased results in weight-loss. However, it can be tremendously life-sustaining to people who suffer from coeliac disease or have allergies or sensitivity to gluten. A gluten-free diet has proved to be extremely crucial for those who suffer from coeliacs, an autoimmune or inflammatory disorder, in which their body cannot properly digest foods that contain gluten. Since the gluten isn't recognized by the body's immune system, it actually attacks the intestinal tract and can cause severe damage to your body.

People who are unaware of their sensitivity to gluten are at a high risk of having permanent damage caused to their bodies, as well as nutrient-loss, since their digestive tract is no longer able to absorb nutrients from their food properly.

Gluten may very well be the cause of various "mysterious" digestive issues you may be having, such as gas, bloating and sluggishness. An astounding 40% of people carry the HLA-DQ2 and HLA-DQ8 genes, which cause people to be susceptible to gluten-sensitivity. That being said, there is a surprisingly high chance that you may very well be experiencing these digestive issues due to gluten-insensitivity. In this case, eliminating gluten from your diet can greatly improve digestion, increase energy levels and strongly contribute to your overall health and well-being.

Recognizing the symptoms of gluten-intolerance beforehand will greatly reduce the risks of permanent damage to your digestive tract and overall health. Here are some of the symptoms associated with allergies and sensitivity to gluten:

- Gas
- Bloating
- Diarrhea and other digestive issues
- Severe, intractable dandruff
- Itchy rashes
- Foggy brain
- Pounding headaches
- Pins and needles sensation
- Irritability
- Depression or Anxiety

If you have coeliacs disease allergies to gluten, consuming it can lead to many unwanted illnesses and health concerns. A review in the New England Journal of Medicine listed 55 diseases that can potentially be caused by consuming gluten. These include osteoporosis, irritable bowel disease, inflammatory bowel disease, anemia, cancer, fatigue, canker sores, rheumatoid arthritis, lupus, multiple sclerosis, and almost every other autoimmune disease.

Gluten can also be linked to a wide array of mental and neurological illnesses such as as schizophrenia, anxiety, dementia, depression, migraines, neuropathy (nerve damage) and autism.

These statistics are especially alarming because 99% of people with gluten sensitivity aren't even aware that they have it, and gluten is one of the biggest staples in our diets.

Gluten is a form of protein that is found in a plethora of foods that we consume regularly, including pizza, bread, pasta, rolls, and almost all processed foods. It is generally found in wheat, barley, rye, spelt, kamut and oats. This means that a large population of individuals with gluten-intolerance are nonchalantly going about their days while consuming these foods as a part of their daily lifestyle - without having a clue about the damages that gluten is detrimentally causing their bodies, on a daily basis.

A recent large study in the Journal of the American Medical Association found that people who were diagnosed, undiagnosed or "latent" with coeliac disease or gluten sensitivity had a higher risk of death, mostly from developing cancer and heart disease - and yet an astounding 99 PERCENT of the people who suffer from coeliac disease or gluten sensitivity don't even know it.

Should you completely eliminate gluten from your diet or simply reduce your gluten intake?

If you suffer from coeliac disease, there is absolutely no question in completely removing gluten from your diet, as a gluten-free diet is critically life-sustaining and crucial to your ultimate health and well-being. However, if you merely suffer from gluten-sensitivity, you can try limiting your intake of gluten-containing foods to maybe a few times a week, to see how your body reacts. If the digestive issues persist, you can further reduce your gluten-intake. If you feel that you have the best results when completely eliminating gluten from your diet, this just might be the way to go. Everyone is different, and some may have a more heightened level of gluten-sensitivity than others, including an increased amount/severity of adverse reactions. So it's a good idea to balance out the pros and cons until you see what works best for you.

Chapter 5: What is Coeliac Disease?

Coeliac disease is a genetic digestive and autoimmune disorder in which an individual is extremely sensitive to gluten. Someone who suffers from coeliac disease will have damage caused to the lining of the small intestine if they consume foods containing gluten. Damage in the small intestine results in a difficulty for the body to properly absorb enough nutrients from food, especially calcium, iron, fat and folate.

The body's immune system is designed to play a major role in protecting it from foreign invaders. If you have coeliac disease, your body recognizes gluten as one of these foreign invaders and produces antibodies to fight it, while attacking the lining of your small intestines. This results in inflammation, as well as damage to the villi, the hair-like structures on the lining of the small intestine. Nutrients are generally absorbed by the villi, which means that if the villi is damaged the body will not be able to properly absorb these nutrients from food.

Symptoms of Coeliac Disease:

Here is a list of symptoms that are associated with coeliac disease. Keep in mind that symptoms vary among different people who suffer from this disease.

- Digestive issues such as abdominal discomfort or pain, gas, bloating, diarrhea, pale stools and weight loss

- Growth and developmental problems in children

- A severe skin rash dermatitis herpetiformis (DH)

- Pale stools with foul odor

- Anemia (caused by iron deficiency) that does not respond to iron therapy

- Liver and biliary tract disorders

- Fatigue

- Tooth discoloration or loss of enamel

- Unexplained infertility or recurring miscarriages

- Delayed puberty

- Joint pain

- Weight loss

Diagnosis of Coeliac Disease:

Coeliac disease is commonly diagnosed with blood tests. A doctor may also need to examine a small piece of tissue from your small intestine to determine whether you have coeliac disease. The treatment for coeliac disease (and gluten sensitivity) is a gluten-free diet.

Chapter 6: Why Gluten-Free Flours are Better than Commonly Used Wheat Flour!

Although giving up gluten may seem like a big loss, it actually has many favorable advantages in the flour department. Gluten-free flours are actually much more nutrient-dense, as opposed to processed white flour, which is completely devoid of nutrients. That being said, you'll be getting a good dose of vitamins and nutrients from your starches that you most likely would not be getting from a gluten filled diet.

When it comes to the flour department, a gluten-free diet is definitely a blessing in disguise!

Here are some great gluten-free flours that are packed with nutrients to keep you healthy, and won't give you the gluten-intolerance symptoms! (Thank goodness).

1). Amaranth flour

Amaranth flour is extremely high in nutritional value, and is higher in protein than most commonly used grains (with the exception of quinoa). It has a nearly perfect balance of amino acids, and is also very high in essential vitamins and minerals like iron, manganese, phosphorus and magnesium, as well as fiber. It also contains a high content of calcium (especially important in a gluten-free diet!), pantothenic acid, potassium, protein, vitamin b6, zinc. Unlike most grains it contains vitamin C, and is also high in vitamin A.

2). Garbanzo Bean Flour

This particular four is commonly referred to as Dahl flour or channa Dahl in India, and is known in England, as well as the most of Europe as gram flour. This highest quality garbanzo bean flour comes from India and is golden in color with no brown specs of skin. This flour is especially great for baking gluten-free desserts - check out our garbanzo bean chocolate cake recipe under our dessert recipes section of this book!

3). Quinoa Flour

Quinoa is gluten-free nutrient goldmine! Recent studies have shown that quinoa contains many anti-inflammatory phytonutrients, making it an amazing superfood that should indeed be a staple in everyone's diet - regardless of being gluten-free or not! Quinoa is also high in protein and fiber, which make it a whole lot more filling than your typical grains, and is also high in heart-healthy omega-3s, packing in an extra punch of benefits for your ticker! Score!

This little gluten-free gem can be used for everything - you can use quinoa to to make baked goods, breakfast bars and parfaits, and savory dinners that your whole family will enjoy!

4). Chia Flour

Like amaranth flour, chia flour is also extremely nutritious. This flour is made up of ground chia seeds, which have been labeled a superfood! Chia flour is packed with Omega-3, protein, calcium and fiber, making it an impressively superior alternative to processed wheat flour, which is useless in the nutrient-department.

Fun fact: Chia seeds are known as "nature's rocket fuel" to many super-athletes and sportspeople, who also use it as an energy enhancement during physical activity, as well as sports events!

5. Lupin Flour

Lupin flour is made from a legume that is in the same family as peanuts. Lupin flour is also an excellent baking choice because it's a great source of both protein and fiber. However, since it's in the same family as peanuts, it carries the same protein that causes allergic reactions/anaphylaxis to peanuts and legumes, and therefore is unsuitable for those who have allergies to peanuts and legumes (this also includes soybeans).

6). Soya Flour

This particular flour is high in protein and has a distinct nutty taste to it. Generally, soya flour isn't used on its own in gluten-free baking, but can be used in conjunction with other gluten-free flours (tapioca flour, for example) as an excellent thickener and flavor enhancer. However, since soya flour is high in fat, it should be stored carefully in a cool, dark environment to prevent it from turning rancid. You can also store this flour in your refrigerator to prevent it from going bad.

7). Tapioca Flour

Tapioca flour is made from the cassava plant and is an excellent addition to any wheat-free kitchen! This flour is great because it adds chewiness and is also a good thickener, making it an excellent wheat flour replacement! Tapioca flour is fairly resilient and can be stored at room temperature.

8). Teff Flour

This flour is made up of ground teff, which is a grain that is about the size of a poppy seed. Teff is predominantly grown in Ethiopia and Eritrea, and can thrive in many climates. Teff's history can be traced back thousands of years, to the ancient civilizations of Abyssinia. It has a delicious yet mild nutty flavor, and also provides an incredible punch of health benefits. Teff is an excellent source of vitamin C, which is a nutrient that isn't commonly found in grains. It also contains an excellent balance of amino acids, and is a great source source of protein, calcium and iron. In fact, it contains the same amount of calcium found in half a cup of cooked spinach. Teff is also high in resistant starch, which is a newly discovered type of fiber that is shown to benefit blood-sugar management, weight control and colon health.

Teff flour can be used to make a wide assortment of baked goods, including pie crusts, cookies, muffins and breads. It can also be boiled or steamed and eaten whole as a side dish or even a main course!

So with all of the amazing, nutrient rich gluten-free flours that are out there, why would you miss nutrient-devoid, useless and processed wheat flour?!

Chapter 7: GF Dining - Tips for Dining Out while on a Gluten-Free Diet

So you're on a gluten-free diet now, and your family wants to go out to eat at a restaurant - what on earth do you do?

A gluten-free diet should never ever have to prevent you from enjoying a meal with your family members, friends and loved ones at a restaurant. This is why we've provided some greatly useful tips for dining out while gluten-free.

Gluten-Free Dining out Tips:

1). If possible, try and go to restaurants that offer a gluten-free menu.

The most trustworthy restaurants have certification or training through a coeliac support group, and are knowledgable about important aspects like the issue of cross-contamination (when otherwise gluten-free foods are exposed to and contaminated by foods that contain gluten).

2). Ask the Server Important Questions

Don't be afraid of sounding annoying when it comes to asking the server/waiter questions! It's important for your own health to inform the restaurant server about your special diet needs.

Tell the server that that you have coeliac or gluten intolerance and need to avoid everything (including seasonings, sauces and dips!) containing gluten. Tell them that this includes wheat, barley, rye, most oats, flour, breading, soy or teriyaki sauce, and seasonings that contain flour as an ingredient.

3). Ask the Server about Preparation!

This is an important one. Ask the server about how the food's been prepared, as this can cross-contaminate foods that would otherwise be gluten-free. Here are some specific questions you should ask the server regarding this matter:

- Are the French fries made in a specific dedicated fryer?
- Are all of the gluten-free foods prepared in a separate area dedicated to being gluten free using dedicated pots, pans and utensils?
- Is the grill cleaned before the gluten-free food is prepared?

4). If unsure about the restaurant's gluten-free menu, order "safe" foods.

If you are unsure about the restaurant's validity in terms of the gluten-free menu, or they're unable to give satisfactory answers to your important questions, order the items that are least likely to be cross-contaminated. For example, rather than ordering yourself fried potatoes, opt for a plain baked potato instead. It would be also a wise idea to ask for the grill/pan to be cleaned before any meat, seafood or poultry is prepared. Plain & fresh fruit and veggies are great to order as side-dishes to make your meal more filling.

5). Take advantage of online gluten-free restaurant websites and apps.

There a number of websites and smart phone apps that are greatly helpful in locating restaurants that meet your gluten-free dietary needs.

Gluten-Free Restaurant Locating Websites and Apps:

Allergy Eats - This site provides online information about gluten-free and allergy-free restaurants and is searchable by location.

Find Me Gluten Free - This site provides online information about gluten-free restaurants nearby and is searchable by address. You can also only search for restaurants that offer a SPECIFIC gluten-free menu. Talk about convenient!

Gluten Free Passport - This site provides online information that is searchable by categories like fast food chains, ethnic cuisines and GF menus.

Gluten Free Travel Site - This site is perfect for when you're traveling! It provides handy online information about gluten-free restaurants located in your area, and is searchable by country, state and zip code.

Other helpful restaurant locating sites include Celiac Travel and Triumph Dining.

These phone apps/websites will help you plan ahead and will make your life a whole lot easier!

Chapter 8: 8 Tips to Make your Gluten-Free Lifestyle Much Easier

Although converting to a gluten-free diet may seem like a hassle at first, there are a number of things that you can do to make your foodie-life go much smoother. We've included a handy list of things you can do to make life easier while on a gluten-free diet.

1). Plan Ahead

Planning ahead will make things less stressful while on a GF diet because you won't have to spend extra time trying to figure out what you can have for lunch right now. Instead, you'll be prepared. It's helpful to make a weekly menu and plan what meals you'll be having.

2). Eat Whole Foods

Although it may be tempting to always rely on packaged gluten-free foods, you should try your hardest to eat as many whole foods as you can while you're on a gluten-free diet. Packaged gluten-free foods are convenient, but they're also processed which means they're not as high in nutrients as quality whole foods that are naturally gluten-free.

3). Make a Big Batch of Soup

Soup is filling, and you can make a big batch of it that will last you several days. Instead of trying to muster up a gluten-free meal whenever you're hungry, you'll have a soup conveniently waiting for you in the fridge.

4). Cook Ahead and Freeze Meals

Cook large batches of gluten-free meals, and freeze the uneaten portions. This is a convenient way to have fully-cooked and delicious meals ready for the entire family already, and will eliminate the need to spend an hour in the kitchen cooking dinner. Just grab the frozen meal, pop it in the microwave, and voila! Dinner is served.

5). Purchase Separate Utensils to Avoid Cross-Contamination

This is an important one. For some people, even a tiny amount of gluten will lead to them experiencing symptoms - this can happen by eating otherwise gluten-free foods that were contaminated by a gluten-exposed toaster or utensils. Buy a separate toaster and utensils, and place them in a designated area to avoid cross-contamination.

6). Eat Foods that are in Season

Try to always purchase foods that are in season. These foods travel less far to reach your grocery store, and therefore are cheaper.

7). Invest in a Good Vacuum Food Sealer.

This will allow your food to stay fresh for a longer period of time, preventing it from going to waste.

8). Invest in a Bread-maker

Investing in a bread maker will allow you to save lots of money in the long run, because you'll be able to make your own bread (and get creative mixing various flours!) instead of spending boatloads of cash on pricey prepackaged gluten-free breads. Score!

Chapter 9: Kids on a Gluten-Free Diet: Tips to Make Life Easier

Having kids who require being on a gluten-free diet can often be quite stressful. Kids are notorious for being picky eaters, and it can often be rather difficult to find gluten-free foods, particularly school lunches that they'll actually enjoy.

This is why we've decided to compile a list of kid-friendly meal options that are not only gluten-free, but also healthy, filling, nourishing and delicious! This will help reduce complaints from your picky little fussy eaters, and result in them licking their fingers instead!

GLUTEN-FREE SCHOOL LUNCH IDEAS FOR THE KIDDOS

Here are some great ideas for gluten-free packed lunches:

- Leftover gluten-free pizza slices
- Peanut butter and jelly sandwiches on gluten free bread or in between 2 gluten-free pancakes.

- Tuna or chicken salad sandwiches on gluten free bread. Tip: For softer "sandwiches", use gluten-free pancakes instead of sandwich bread!

- Homemade corn tortilla burritos (you can really get creative here! Use beans for added protein and fiber!)

- Fried rice with chicken and veggies. You can also use quinoa as a healthier and more protein-filled option!

- Baked potato in a thermos - add favorite toppings, wrap in aluminum foil and slide into the thermos to keep it warm!

- Turkey and cheese roll ups.

- Leftover dinner in a thermos.

- Hardboiled eggs.

- Deviled eggs

- Gluten-free English muffin pizzas

- Chicken or beef kabobs (cut them up into cubes and pierce them onto a wooden kabob skewer)

- Martha Stewart's Gluten-Free Corn Tortilla Crusted Chicken Tenders (because kids love chicken tenders!) Recipe below:

Ingredients:

- 10 corn tortillas, roughly torn
- Coarse salt and ground pepper

- 1/4 cup all-purpose flour
- 1 cup buttermilk
- 12 chicken tenders (about 1 1/2 pounds total)
- 2 cups vegetable oil
- 3 tablespoons grainy mustard
- 3 tablespoons honey

Directions:

In a food processor, pulse tortillas until mixture is similar to coarse meal. Season with salt and pepper to taste and transfer to a medium sized bowl.

Put flour on a plate and pour the buttermilk into a shallow dish. Rub chicken in flour, shaking off any excess flour. Coat in buttermilk, letting excess drip off, and then roll your chicken in tortilla crumbs, pressing gently to adhere. Transfer to a large baking sheet.

In a large nonstick skillet, heat oil over medium heat. Cook chicken until it is fully cooked throughout and crust is golden, flipping once - this should take about 12 minutes. Transfer to paper towels or a wire rack over a rimmed baking sheet to drain. In a small bowl, stir together mustard and honey until the mixture has become well combined. Serve the chicken tenders with honey mustard dip.

Tip: Serve the chicken tenders with French fries (make sure they're gluten free) for a traditional kid-favorite meal!

KID FRIENDLY GLUTEN-FREE SNACKS

Finding the appropriate kid-friendly snacks can often be difficult and seem like a major task when you have a child with a gluten allergy. Virtually, it seems like all convenient kid-friendly snacks have gluten hidden in them (crackers, tortilla chips, muffins, cookies, granola, cereal bars, etc).

However, there's no need for you to lose hope! We've decided to compile a convenient list of yummy snacks that are not only gluten-free but also kid-friendly, and great for adults, too! These snacks satisfy virtually every craving, whether you're in the mood for something fruity or veggie, crunchy, creamy, sweet, salty or chocolaty!

- Fresh Fruit and Veggies (can be dipped in nut butters)
- Dried Fruit
- Fruit Leather (a healthier version of a fruit roll up!)
- Fruit and Cheese Kabobs
- Apples with Peanut Butter
- Applesauce
- Olives
- Strawberry and Homemade Whipped Cream
- Celery Sticks with Cream Cheese or Peanut Butter

- Bananas with Peanut Butter and Raisins
- Kale Chips
- Flavorful Homemade Potato Chips with Ranch Dip (Recipe Below!)
- Hummus (makes a great dip for almost everything! I like using it as a healthy dip for baby carrots or bell pepper slices).
- Grain Free Crackers
- Gluten-free Dark Chocolate
- Rice Cakes
- Gluten-Free Gelatin Cups
- Popcorn
- Lemon/Lime Homemade Gluten Free Gelatin (the kids will love this!)

Ingredients:

- 3 Tbsp gelatin, granulated (3 packets)
- 3/4 cup healthiest sweetener of your choice
- 12 scoops stevia extract
- 1 1/2 cups boiling filtered water
- 3 cups cold water (divided)
- 1 1/8 cup lemon or lime juice (or use some of both for Lemon Lime Gelatin!)

- 1/2 teaspoon grated rind (optional. Use lemon rind for lemon gelatin–lime for lime.)

Directions:

1). Soften the gelatin by soaking it in 1 1/2 cups of cold water - this will take a few minutes.

2). Add boiling water and stir until gelatin has become dissolved.

3). Add the rest of the ingredients (including the other 1 1/2 cups cold water), and stir the mixture until thoroughly blended.

4). Pour into 2 8×8 baking pans.

5). Refrigerate until set. Enjoy!

Homemade Potato Chips & Ranch Dip

Ingredients:

- 2 medium potatoes
- 1 TBSP olive oil
- salt and pepper

Directions:

1). Wash the potatoes and peel off the skin, if desired. Slice thinly - not too thin, but not too thick either (think of your ideally sized potato chips). Drizzle olive oil over the slices. Grease a cookie sheet with some more olive oil and lay the slices over a single layer.

2). Sprinkle salt and pepper over potato slices to taste. Bake at 400 degrees F for 20 minutes, or until edges are browned.

3). Optional: You can also make things interesting and add your favorite flavors (think flavored potato chips!) I like using spices like garlic, dill and chili powder!

Ranch Dip:

Ingredients:

- 1/2 cup Greek or strained yogurt
- 2 oz cream cheese, softened
- 1/4 cup heavy cream mixed with 1 tsp lemon juice
- 1 tsp dried parsley
- 1/2 teaspoon dried dill-weed
- 1/2 teaspoon sea salt
- 1/4 teaspoon ground black pepper
- 1 clove garlic, minced

Directions:

Combine all of the ingredients and mix together. Dip your potato chips in it and enjoy!

Chapter 10: Benefits of a Gluten-Free Diet in Children with Autism

A gluten-free diet has also proved to have extremely favorable benefits in children who have Autism. There have many been cases in which severely autistic children (some of which who can't even speak) have showed significant behavioral improvements as a result of a gluten-free diet. In fact, the children's behavioral problems have been reduced so drastically that they now speak and behave like non-autistic children. Yes, they still have some Autism-related behavioral problems, but not nearly as much as they initially had before they switched to a gluten-free diet.

Chapter 11: Gluten Intolerance VS Lactose Intolerance

It's surprisingly common for people with a gluten-allergy to mistake it for lactose-intolerance, or vice versa. This can often be a tricky and confusing misconception, due to the fact that these two very different conditions have nearly identical symptoms.

Understanding the differences between lactose intolerance and gluten sensitivity can be very important, and in some cases absolutely crucial. For example, if someone who actually has coeliac disease believes they are lactose intolerant, they'll be more than likely to cause significant damage to their bodies with their eating habits, since they wouldn't be treating their condition with the one absolutely necessary treatment that their bodies require: completely abstaining from any gluten-containing foods. This is why it's incredibly important to have an understanding about the differences of gluten intolerance and lactose intolerance, and to know how to distinguish between the two.

Lactose Intolerance:

Lactose intolerance is generally what happens when a person is unable to digest lactose, which is a naturally occurring milk sugar. In order to digest lactose, an individual's body needs lactase, which is a naturally occurring enzyme. If a person's body is either unable to produce this enzyme, or not enough of it, consuming dairy products will instead cause the lactose to form a hydrogen gas in the colon, which will lead the person to experience digestive symptoms like gas, nausea and bloating (the same symptoms that occur in those with an intolerance to gluten).

Lactose intolerance affects a large amount of people. For example, an astounding 30 - 50 million of Americans are affected by it. However, it is not an allergy and should not be confused with a gluten allergy or celiac. It is far less common to have a gluten allergy or even celiac disease than it is to be lactose-intolerant.

A primary aspect that sets lactose intolerance apart from the zero-tolerance-for-gluten-whatsoever disease, otherwise known as coeliac disease is the fact that consuming lactose if you're lactose intolerant will not cause permanent damage to your digestive tract, and the symptoms will only occur as a temporary aftermath of recently consuming lactose.

People who are diagnosed with lactose intolerance generally avoid consuming lactose for the sole purpose of preventing gastrointestinal discomfort related symptoms. What separates this from celiac disease is the fact that celiac-sufferers must always avoid gluten (at ALL costs), because this is the only way to treat their disease, as well as prevent permanent intestinal damage and further diseases.

Unfortunately, celiac disease and gluten allergies are commonly overlooked and often mistaken as lactose intolerance - that is, until the person begins to develop more advanced symptoms. At this point, there may have already been significant and irreversible damage done to the person's body that would have been 100% preventable, had they eliminated gluten from their diet.

This is why it's important to be aware of the important key aspects that differentiate a gluten allergy/celiac disease from lactose intolerance and adjust your diet accordingly.

Getting an accurate diagnosis requires being medically tested - this will determine whether you're lactose-intolerant, or have coeliac disease. However, many people with coeliac disease also experience lactose-intolerance as a result of their disease. Therefore, if you have both coeliac disease and lactose-intolerance, eliminating gluten from your diet will most likely eliminate the lactose intolerance as well.

Chapter 12: Can Coeliac Disease Affect the Brain?

Did you know that there has been medical evidence indicating that gluten can negatively impact the brains of those who suffer from coeliacs, causing complex brain conditions such as seizures, hallucinations, and even autism?

Here is one particular documented medical case that supports this astounding new information regarding coeliac disease being linked to various complex brain conditions:

When Dr. Andre H. Lagrange, a neurologist at Vanderbilt University in Nashville discovered ominous white spots on a patient's brain scan, he first assumed that these white spots were an indication of either an infection or lymphoma (a type of cancer). The patient was also complaining about having unexplained ongoing seizures. However, when multiple tests on the patient had ruled out both of these possibilities, Dr. Lagrange turned to the 30-something-year-old patient's mother, who insisted that the man was continuing to suffer from seizures (despite taking various anti-epilepsy drugs) that were accompanied by consistent spells of constipation and diarrhea.

The man's strange symptoms had prompted Dr. Lagrange to conduct a series of various tests on the frustrated patient, including multiple antibody tests, as well as an intestinal biopsy.

The test results were in, and finally provided answers explaining the cause of the man's unpleasant symptoms: the tests had indicated that the patient had coeliac disease, an autoimmune disorder triggered by gluten proteins. Here's something quite intriguing about this case: once the man removed gluten from his diet, his seizures quickly stopped, and the brain lesions gradually disappeared!

According to Dr. Lagrange, once the coeliac-diagnosed patient completely eliminated gluten from his diet, he made a "nearly complete recovery".

This particular case is a prime example of why many medical professionals believe that coeliac disease often extends beyond the gut and can affect other organs, such as the brain, like the case with this particular coeliac patient. According to Dr. Lagrange, coeliac disease can lead to many complex conditions of the brain, including seizures, hallucinations, psychotic breaks, and even regressive autism. Although the specific cause of this remains unclear, there have been numerous cases which have proven that there is, in fact a link between the intestinal tract and the central nervous system in those who suffer from coeliac disease. In all of these cases, recovery was not a result of drugs directed at the brain. It was only achieved when the coeliac sufferer removed gluten completely from their diet.

These medical studies are important warnings about how critical and health-sustaining it is to stick to a diet that is completely free of gluten when you have coeliac disease.

Chapter 13: The story of Jess Madden: a Doctor and Coeliac Patient

Dr. Jess Madden has been experiencing both sides of medicine since her coeliac diagnosis in 2010. She is both a neonatologist and coeliac patient, carrying the dual identity of simultaneously being the doctor and the patient.

After years of suffering the unpleasant symptoms of undiagnosed coeliac disease, she finally was given a diagnoses in 2010. Like most other newly diagnosed coeliac patient, she had a lot to learn at the beginning of her gluten-free journey. Being in the patient's position has opened Dr. Madden's eyes to how much room for improvement there is in terms of doctor-patient communication, as well as determining the correct diagnosis when it comes to coeliac disease.

Apart from being a doctor and a coeliac patient, she is also an blogger, and shares her personal experiences with managing her disease on her blog, "The Patient Celiac".

Dr. Madden has recently done an interview with the Gluten Free Living magazine, in which she has described her everyday life as a coeliac patient and a neonatologist.

When asked what her mornings are typically like, and what she eats for breakfast, this was Dr. Jess Madden's reply:

"I either eat a bowl of gluten-free oatmeal and some fruit, or I make a smoothie and use whatever I can find in the fridge. It's usually kale, berries, almond milk, and I'll throw yogurt in or almond butter. I drink a lot of coffee. Usually, it's pretty hectic getting three of my four kids and my niece off to school between eating breakfast, getting dressed and making sure they have their homework. I am getting ready for work, too. Luckily, I wear scrubs to work. The kids are out the door by 7:45 a.m. I leave the house at 8:00 a.m., and my workday starts at 8:30 a.m."

When asked by Gluten Free Living what an average day is usually like for her, this was Dr. Jess Madden's response:

"I work in a neonatal intensive care unit (NICU). From 8:30 a.m. until about 2 p.m. we do what's called "rounding." I go "bed side" and see every baby in the unit. I examine them, make a plan for the day for each one, update the family and write a daily progress note. It's broken up because if there is a high-risk delivery or a premature baby being born, we leave the NICU to help out. I do consultations, and then I make a lot of phone calls. Until I leave at 4:30 p.m., I do administrative work, catch up on emails, or I start to read articles on celiac disease. I work night shifts about six times a month and that's when I work on my blog.

Most of my writing is done at 1:00 a.m. I'll post to my blog at 3 in the morning and the same with my Facebook posts and tweets on Twitter. The nurses I work with in the NICU are so used to hearing about everything I'm writing about. They have been very involved in the process, too. Some of them help me proofread posts."

"When I work at night, it's not the typical day I just described. On those days, I spend a lot of my time with my 2-year-old. I use those days for catching up on life. The next day I sleep during the day."

When asked what she usually has for lunch, this was Dr. Jess' response:

"Lunch is usually leftovers from dinner the night before. I am really fortunate right now that my husband is doing all of the cooking. If I forget to bring lunch, we have a doctors' lounge and one of the members of the food services team also has celiac disease and will leave me gluten-free food. Sometimes I get a salad and hard boiled eggs."

When asked if there was anything surprising in particular about her typical day, this is what Dr. Jess Madden had to say:

"Things can get really hectic at a moment's notice in neonatology. I never know when a woman is going to come in and deliver a premature baby. It's an environment where things can change really rapidly.

You can have a baby who is fine and gets really sick all of a sudden."

When asked what a typical dinner was for her, this was Dr. Jess Madden's reply:

"We are a totally gluten-free home. Our typical rotation includes chicken or seafood, enchiladas and pizza."

This was Dr. Jess Madden's response when she was asked what her favorite part of the day was:

"My favorite parts of the day are when we eat dinner together as a family and then the time between dinner and getting my kids tucked into bed."

When Dr. Jess Madden was asked how it was like to reverse roles and go from doctor to patient, this is how she answered:

"Other than when I gave birth, it's really the first time I have ever been in the patient's position. That's been really eye opening about how much room there is for improvement in patient/doctor communication and in terms of determining difficult diagnoses, as celiac disease can often be. I think it has made me much more empathetic with patients and their families. My blog's name is a play on words because I try to be patient with things, but I have a tendency to not be. In terms of healing, I do have to have patience."

(Source: Gluten Free Living magazine)

What makes Dr. Jess Madden's blog so special is how it allows you to become exposed to the personal experiences and valid medical advice from an actual doctor - a coeliac patient who can share details about this disease from a medical professional's point of view.

Dr. Madden's blog, "The Patient Celiac" is a wonderfully inspiring, as well as highly informative and personable blog that shares with you the everyday life of a coeliac patient who also happens to be a doctor. This doctor/coeliac patient's blog is filled with plenty of valuable, interesting, and inspiring information that will make a coeliac patient feel like they aren't alone in managing their unique condition.

Chapter 14: Your Guide to a Gluten-Free Meal Plan

Now that we've established how important it is to completely remove gluten from your diet if you suffer from coeliac disease or sensitivity to gluten, let's move on to a helpful guide that will let you know everything about maintaining a healthy, nutritious (and delicious!) gluten-free diet and lifestyle.

Grocery shopping for gluten-free foods:

When shopping at your local supermarket for gluten-free foods, it's important to keep in mind that gluten is hidden in a wide array of foods - not just in the obvious culprits like wheat bread and pasta. Here's an included list of foods that contain gluten.

Gluten-Containing Foods to Avoid:

Barley, barley malt/extract, bran, bulgur, couscous, durum, einkorn, emmer, farina, faro, graham flour, kamut, matzo flour/meal, orzo, panko, rye, seitan, semolina, spelt, triticale, udon, wheat, wheat bran, wheat germ, wheat starch.

Commonly Overlooked Foods that Contain Gluten:

Ales, beer and lagers, breading, brown rice syrup, coating mix, communion wafers, croutons, candy, luncheon meat, broth, pasta, roux, sauces, soup base, stuffing, self-basting poultry, imitation bacon/seafood, soy sauce, marinades, thickeners, herbal supplements, prescription medications and over the counter medications, lipstick, gloss and balms, play-dough.

This doesn't by any means imply that you should stop taking your medication without first consulting your doctor. This only means that you should be mindful of the fact that there are many, MANY sources of gluten. It also means that if you have gluten-sensitive young children, make sure that they don't eat any of their play-dough during playtime! (This also goes for every child - gluten sensitive or not!)

ENJOYING GLUTEN-FREE MEALS

Although it may seem frustrating at first to have to give up your favorite gluten-filled foods, don't lose hope! There are many gluten-free alternatives available for the foods you love. The majority of supermarkets (particularly health food stores) carry a wide variety of gluten-free versions of your favorite meals, including bread, pizza, pasta, burritos, macaroni and cheese, lasagna, and many more! There are even many gluten-free desserts available, such as chocolate cake and ice cream! Just look for a "gluten-free" label and begin stocking up on all of your favorite foods - including desserts!

A popular brand that offers a wide variety of gluten-free dishes (over 125!) is Amy's Kitchen. Amy's Kitchen meals can be found in the frozen food aisle at many grocery stores. Not only are these meals gluten-free, they're also organic and GMO-free, providing you with additional health benefits.

Amy's Kitchen is a family-owned, privately held company that was founded in 1987 by CEO Andy Berliner and his wife, Rachel Berliner. The company was named after their daughter, Amy and has been dedicated to providing customers with many gluten-free alternatives to their traditional favorites, like pizza and macaroni cheese, as well as a variety of ethnic-style foods, such as Asian Noodle Stir-fry, Thai Red Curry and Mexican Casserole Bowl.

GLUTEN-FREE CARBOHYDRATES AND STARCHES

Many people mistakenly assume that a gluten-free lifestyle will inevitably prevent them from eating energy boosting carbohydrates. Rest assured, this is not the case. There is still a wide variety of starchy carbohydrates that are perfectly acceptable options while on a gluten-free diet. These include:

- Rice
- Soy
- Beans
- Polenta
- Potatoes (including sweet potatoes)

- Buckwheat (kasha)
- Millet
- Corn tortillas
- Gluten-free breads/pasta/baking mixes
- Flax
- Amaranth
- Arrowroot
- Sorghum
- Tapioca
- Quinoa
- Chia
- Teff
- Yucca

While on a gluten-free diet, you can still enjoy a wide variety of delicious and satisfying foods, such as beef, poultry, seafood, eggs, fruits and vegetables, nuts, beans and legumes and dairy. However, while fresh and frozen fruits and veggies are naturally gluten-free, it's important to be cautious and read the labels of processed and dried fruits and vegetables, as well as packaged frozen potatoes, since these options aren't always gluten-free.

Chapter 15: Gluten-Free on a Budget

While a gluten-free diet is extremely beneficial as well as crucial for those suffering from coeliac disease or gluten sensitivity, it can also be quite costly. Here are some tips on living gluten-free while on a budget.

Buy naturally gluten-free pantry items on sale.

Many people on a gluten-free diet focus mainly on buying packaged "gluten-free" labeled foods. However, it can be difficult to maintain a budget when the $7.95 gluten-free baking mixes, and $6.99 gluten free breads begin to exponentially add up. That being said, stock up on naturally gluten-free pantry items on sale. These include beans, rice, canned vegetables, canned pumpkin, quinoa, tapioca and buckwheat groats (also known as kasha).

Make your own snacks instead of opting for prepackaged ones.

Making your own snacks, such as hummus and corn tortilla chips will provide you with twice the amount of snack foods, for half the price of buying pricey, gluten-free packaged snacks.

Grow your own vegetable garden!

A great way to save plenty of money while on a gluten-free diet is by growing your own vegetable garden. Eliminating the need to make weekly trips to the produce aisle will significantly help you save money, and in turn, allow you to afford those delicious and convenient gluten-free packaged meals and desserts, especially if you have dessert-loving, gluten-sensitive children.

Chapter 16: Incredibly Healthy Gluten Free Super-Foods

Incredibly Healthy Gluten-Free Super-Foods

Many people view a gluten-free diet as merely an inconvenient and restrictive loss that greatly limits your food-intake options, making life boring, bland and ultimately challenging. Not true! Now that you have a gluten-free lifestyle, you can actually view it is an advantage - an opportunity to replace unhealthy calorie-laden, starchy foods with little to zero nutritional value (ahem - greasy buns, artery clogging pizza and pastries) with naturally healthy and delicious whole foods that pack on a wide array of health-boosting properties, and will ultimately benefit all aspects of your health!

You can view a gluten-free diet as an amazing opportunity to fuel your body with a good dose of much-needed nutrients, which in turn will improve many aspects of your physical health (we've listed them below!), energy levels and general well-being by filling up on plenty of colorful super-foods! The great part about a gluten-free diet is that it doesn't limit you from eating any of your favorite fresh fruits and vegetables! Instead of seeing your gluten-free lifestyle as a limitation, see it as a wonderful opportunity to colorfully expand your palate with nature's amazingly healthy and nutritious super-foods!

Here is a list of naturally gluten-free super-foods that you should definitely include into your gluten-free lifestyle, and what makes them so incredibly good for us.

1). Apples

There's definitely a reason for the age-old, popular saying, "an apple a day keeps the doctor away"! Did you know that an apple a day can also keep Alzheimer's away? Eating an apple each day will keep you sharp and alert, as it will prevent deterioration in brain function! Apples are packed with an impressively high content of flavonoids and polyphenols, which are both powerful antioxidants that help reduce your risk of lung cancer and bladder cancer. These antioxidants also fight aging, which help your skin have a youthful and vibrant appearance! In addition, eating an apple every day has also shown to lower cholesterol!

Did you know that apples can also help you lose weight more effectively? An intriguing study has shown that women who ate 3 apples a day had significantly better weight-loss results than those who didn't!

2). Asparagus

Asparagus contains many health-boosting properties! It contains asparagine, an active amino acid that helps your body get rid of excess water (it is a natural diuretic). Asparagus is also known to have anti-inflammatory properties, and is therefore helpful in easing the symptoms of rheumatoid arthritis and asthma. This handy little green vegetable has also shown to have a positive impact on irritability, fatigue and depression, as well as in stabilizing blood-sugar levels (great for diabetics).

3). Bananas

Bananas are great energy boosters, and make a perfectly delicious pre-workout snack! Bananas are an excellent source of vitamin B6 and vitamin C, as well as fiber, magnesium and potassium. The potassium found in bananas is shown to regulate blood pressure, which can help prevent heart disease and stroke.

Bananas are also great for those who have gastrointestinal issues as a result of celiac disease because they are very easy to digest, and won't put strain on your body's digestive process.

Bonus Fact: Did you know that bananas contain serotonin and norepinephrine which naturally help treat depression?

4). Beet root

Beet root is a wonderful addition to a gluten-free diet, because it offers such an impressively wide variety of health benefits! Consuming this vibrantly colorful, bright purple vegetable will definitely add color to your life!

Beets contain the bio-active agent betaine, which highly supports liver function. They're also an excellent source of folic acid, fiber, manganese, potassium, phosphorus, magnesium, iron and vitamin B6. Beets also contain a powerful antioxidant called betacyanin, which is responsible for giving beets their bright purple color and has been shown to provide protection against certain oxidative-stress relates disorders in humans.

There's also evidence that supports that eating beets can help prevent cancer, particularly skin and lung cancers. Another study has shown that beets contain anti-cancer compounds called nitrosamines, which inhibit the formation of cancer.

Fun Bonus: Did you know that beets are also natural aphrodisiacs? Beets are rich in boron, which naturally increases and benefits the libido, making them great little bedroom-boosters!

"Beetroot definitely beats purple Chanel lipstick."

- Quote by Thas

5). Carrots

Carrots are wonderfully health-boosting orange-colored gems! Carrots contain carotene, which is a chemical that becomes converted to vitamin A by the body, and can help prevent blindness (this is where that common old belief of carrots being good for your peepers comes from!)

However, eyesight isn't the only thing that carrots are good for! Carrots have also been shown to regulate blood sugar, promote colon health, and improve skin by preventing degeneration of cells. Carrots are also a good source of fiber, which helps prevent heart disease.

6). Chili Peppers

Although they are notorious for being quite spicy, chili peppers are also one of nature's healthiest gifts to us!

Chili peppers contain a chemical called capsaicin, which is what gives peppers their flaming-hot trademark characteristic. These spicy little health-boosters are known to contain a plethora of health benefits! They can help protect your heart, lower blood pressure, fight inflammation, and even soothe intestinal diseases.

The capsaicin in chili peppers has also been shown to highly promote weight loss! It is often used as the metabolism-boosting thermogenic ingredient in weight loss supplements, helping you burn fat and lose excess weight!

7). Dates

Dates are an especially wonderful addition to any gluten-free diet! They are incredibly delicious and naturally sweet, and have the chewy consistency that is often sorely missed by those who must steer clear of gluten. Not only are dates amazingly healthy, but they're also a perfectly delicious staple in gluten-free baking!

Dates aid in digestion by helping increase friendly bacteria in your intestines. If you have celiac disease, dates can help restore the healthy bacteria in your gut that is often lost as a result of damage in the intestinal villi.

Dates can also improve your heart health, and even increase your sexual stamina, in addition to being delicious natural desserts!

8). Honeydew

Who needs nutrient-devoid (and not to mention, totally unhealthy) gluten-filled candy when you can have nature's deliciously sweet and refreshingly natural health-boosting candy? In addition to being naturally sweet and mouthwateringly delicious, honeydew also contains a naturally occurring chemical called adenosine, which reduces the risk of cancer and strokes.

9). Avocados

Avocados are great for when you're craving for something that's rich in consistency and flavor, as well as creamy, savory and satisfying! They're also incredibly good for you!

Avocados are high in potassium, and contain monounsaturated fat, which helps regulate blood pressure and keep it at a healthy level. Avocados are also a good source of vitamin K, which help promote health and longevity in the elderly. If you're on a plant-based diet, avocados are also good sources of protein!

10). Broccoli

This super-food is part of the cruciferous vegetable family. Broccoli is known for benefitting the liver by promoting natural detoxification. It is an excellent source of vitamins C and E, which help keep your teeth and gums healthy. Broccoli is also a good source of iron and B-vitamins, which help prevent cancer.

11). Celery

Not only is celery a great, naturally gluten-free snack option that pairs well with peanut butter, as well as cream cheese, but it is also packed with essential health-boosting nutrients that help strengthen your bones and joints! Celery contains high levels of silicon, which helps support and strengthen joints, bones, arteries and connective tissue.

Fun Fact: It has also been said that eating a stalk of celery is just as good for your teeth as brushing them! Who would've thought?!

12). Cranberries

Cranberries are known to boost all aspects of your health and support immune function! These super-berries are high in antioxidants, particularly proanthocyanidins, which are known to benefit overall health. They are also a health-powerhouse, packed with numerous health-boosting vitamins and nutrients that may protect against dental cavities, urinary tract infections, and inflammatory diseases.

13). Kale

It's no wonder that kale is often referred to as a wonder-vegetable! Out of all vegetables, kale contains the highest source of vitamin K, and also helps prevent a number of cancers. Vitamin K has been shown to help with blood-clots and help promote health and longevity in the elderly.

Despite being significantly low in calories, kale is dense with a number of vitamins and nutrients, including calcium, chlorophyll, iron, vitamins A and C, copper, potassium, manganese and phosphorus, as well as compounds which promote eye and skin health.

Kale makes a wonderful addition to a variety of salads and freshly blended health-boosting juices and smoothies.

14). Lemons

Lemons are great for adding flavor to a variety of foods and freshly blended fruit juices, and are high in both vitamin C and anti-inflammatory properties. Lemon and limes also both contain limonene, which studies show may help prevent breast cancer growth. Lemons also contain digestive-aid properties and relieve nausea.

15). Mangoes

These tropical delights contain high contents of vitamin A and vitamin C, which is known to strongly benefit and improve your immune system. Research has also indicated that mangoes help prevent a number of cancers, including colon, breast and prostate cancers, as well as leukemia. Mangoes are also a good source of potassium, which is important in keeping blood pressure and heart rate at healthy levels. In addition, this power-fruit contains various health-boosting flavonoids, including beta-carotene, alpha-carotene, and beta-cryptoxanthin.

16). Onions

Onions have a plethora of health benefits, in addition to adding plenty of flavor to meals. Onions contain a natural occurring chemical that promote bone health while reducing the risk of osteoporosis. They also contain a powerful antioxidant called quercetin, which is an anti-cancer compound that helps prevent cancer, as well as lower blood sugar levels.

17). Papayas

This underrated fruit is amazingly good for us! It contains a powerful anti-cancerous antioxidant that helps prevent cancer, and is also high in vitamins A, C and potassium. Papayas are also packed with healthy enzymes that promote healthy digestion and reduce constipation.

18). Collard Greens

Collard greens are a perfect addition to fresh salads, and contain a high content of chlorophyll, vitamins A, C and E, beta carotene and manganese. Collard greens also contain powerful health-boosting antioxidants that help prevent cancer. Collard greens are also the strongest of greens that lower cholesterol levels.

19). Cucumbers

Cucumbers are very hydrating due to their high water content, and are also very high in potassium and phytosterols which (like collard greens) also help lower cholesterol levels. Consuming cucumbers with their skin (make sure to buy the unwaxed kind) will give you a healthy boost of chlorophyll.

20). Dandelion

Dandelion is very high in vitamin K, and also contains great benefits for your liver and your body's detoxification process. It supports the gall bladder and kidneys as well.

5 INCREDIBLY HEALTHY FLAVOR BOOSTERS:

1). Basil

Basil is a great complimentary spice to many Italian dishes, particularly spaghetti (you can easily whip some up with gluten-free pasta!) and is packed with powerful nutrients. Basil is known to soothe digestive issues, and is a natural antibiotic, antidepressant, and anti-inflammatory agent. It is also a great source of magnesium, which assists in cardiovascular health by promoting healthy blood flow.

2). Cilantro

Cilantro is rich in antioxidants, as well as dietary fiber, which can help lower LDL, or bad cholesterol levels, while raising HDL, or good cholesterol levels. Cilantro is also packed with a plethora of health-boosting vitamins, including folic acid, riboflavin, niacin, vitamin A, beta carotene, vitamin C and vitamin K. Preliminary research also suggests that the coriandrum sativum leaves (a phytonutrient) in cilantro may help manage Alzheimer's disease in many ways, including memory improvement.

3). Cinnamon

Cinnamon is a wonderful way to spice up a variety of desserts, breakfast bars and baked goods while you simultaneously reap great health benefits! Cinnamon is a natural antibiotic, and also helps reduce inflammation while keeping your blood sugar levels healthy.

4). Garlic

In case you haven't heard, garlic delivers incredible benefits to your health! It is a natural antibiotic, antihistamine and diuretic, and helps lower blood sugar and blood cholesterol levels. It's also a powerful immune system booster.

5). Ginger

Ginger contains properties that support digestion, and is also beneficial to your body's natural detoxification system. Ginger has anti-inflammatory and anti-nausea effects, as well.

Chapter 17: Delicious Gluten-Free Recipes (Desserts Included!)

Looking for some delicious, crowd-pleasing, finger-licking-good and ultimately satisfying gluten-free meal ideas? Here is a list of several amazingly delicious gluten-free recipes that are sure to please anyone at your dinner table. These recipes include breakfasts, lunches, dinners, snacks, and even decadent desserts! Some of these recipes, as well as a variety of many other gluten-free recipes can be found on allrecipes.com.

Gluten-Free Recipes

G-Free Banana Pancakes

Ingredients:

- ½ cup milk
- 2 large eggs
- 1½ tbsp butter, melted
- 1 tbsp gluten-free baking powder
- 1 banana
- 1 cup rice flour (or substitute corn, chickpea, or tapioca flour)
- Extra butter for frying pancakes

INSTRUCTIONS:

1) Place all of the liquid ingredients in the bowl of a food processor, and process all of your liquid ingredients together. Slowly add the baking powder, banana, and flour and process until the mixture has gained a smooth consistency.

2) Heat a griddle pan or large frying pan over medium heat, and drop a teaspoon of butter on it. Wait until the butter begins to sizzle, and then pour batter into pan.

3) When bubbles begin to form at the surface, turn the pancakes and continue to fry until golden brown. When finished, place the pancakes on a plate in a warm oven to keep them warm while you make the rest of the pancakes.

(MAKES: 16 pancakes)

Easy and Delicious Breakfast Quinoa

Ingredients:

- ½ cup uncooked quinoa
- 1 cup milk of choice (fat-free suggested)
- 1 tbsp chopped walnuts
- 1 tsp cinnamon
- 1 tbsp almond butter
- ¼ cup fresh blueberries

Directions:

1)   Start off by first placing the quinoa in a fine mesh strainer, and follow by rinsing and draining quinoa.

2)   Combine the quinoa and milk, placing them in a medium-sized to large-sized saucepan. Bring to a boil, and then cover the saucepan, and reduce heat to a gentle simmer. Cook for 10–15 minutes until the milk is absorbed and the quinoa has gained a tender consistency.

3)   Add your walnuts, cinnamon, and almond butter and mix them thoroughly. Let cool. Add fresh blueberries on top.

SERVES: 2

Deliciously Fluffy Gluten-free Pancakes (makes 10 servings)

Ingredients:

- 1 cup rice flour
- 3 tablespoons tapioca flour
- 1/3 cup potato starch
- 4 tablespoons dry buttermilk powder
- 3 teaspoons sugar
- 1 1/2 teaspoon baking powder
- 1/2 teaspoon baking soda
- 1/2 teaspoon salt
- 1/2 teaspoon xanthan gum
- 2 eggs
- 3 tablespoons canola oil
- 2 cups water

Directions:

1)   In a bowl, mix the rice flour, tapioca flour, potato starch, dry buttermilk powder, sugar, baking powder and baking soda. Then, stir in eggs, oil and water and mix well until only a few lumps remain.

2) Heat a large, well-oiled skillet or griddle over medium-high heat. Pour in spoonfuls of the batter onto the skillet and cook until bubbles begin to form. Flip and continue cooking until the pancakes are golden brown. Serve immediately and enjoy!

Breakfast Sausage

Ingredients:

- 2 teaspoons dried sage
- 2 teaspoons salt
- 1 teaspoon ground black pepper
- 1/4 teaspoon dried marjoram
- 1 tablespoon brown sugar
- 1/8 teaspoon crushed red pepper flakes
- 1 pinch ground cloves
- 2 pounds ground pork

Directions:

1) In a small bowl, combine sage, salt, black pepper, crushed red pepper, cloves, brown sugar and marjoram.

2) Place the pork in a large bowl and add the mixed spices to it. Mix well with your hands and form into patties.

3) Sauté the patties in a large skillet over medium-high heat for 5 minutes per side, of until internal pork temperature reaches 160 degrees F (70 degrees C). Enjoy!

Blueberry Oatmeal Breakfast-smoothie

INGREDIENTS:

- ½ cup gluten-free rolled oats
- 1 cup soy milk
- 1 banana, frozen
- ¾ cup fresh or frozen organic blueberries
- 1 tsp honey (optional)
- 4–5 ice cubes (if using fresh blueberries)

INSTRUCTIONS:

Place the oats in a blender and blend for 1–2 minutes until they have been thoroughly ground up into a fine powder. Follow by adding the rest of the ingredients, and blend. Enjoy!

SERVES: 2

Protein Packed Cherry-Quinoa Bars

(Gluten Free Sweet Cherry Quinoa Breakfast/Snack Bars)

INGREDIENTS:

- 1½ cups gluten-free puffed rice cereal
- 1 cup pure rolled oats (make sure they are gluten-free)
- 1 cup cooked quinoa
- ½ cup gluten-free dried cherries, unsweetened
- 1/3 cup sunflower seeds
- 1/3 cup sliced walnuts
- ¼ cup pumpkin seeds
- 2 tbsp flax, ground
- 2 tbsp chia seed, ground
- 1 tsp ground cinnamon
- ½ tsp sea salt
- 1/3 cup sunflower seed butter
- 6 tbsp 100% pure maple syrup

INSTRUCTIONS:

1) Start by first preheating your oven to 325°F. Follow by lining a baking sheet with parchment paper, then set aside.

2) In a large mixing bowl, combine all of the listed ingredients, except for the sunflower seed butter and maple syrup.

3) Mix together your sunflower seed butter and maple syrup. Then heat the mixture in a small saucepan over medium-low heat until it gains a liquefied and smooth consistency.

4) Pour the liquid ingredients over your dry ingredients and mix together until fully combined and everything is coated evenly.

5) Evenly spread your granola out on the parchment-lined baking sheet, onto a thin ¼" layer.

6) Bake the granola in the center of a warmed oven for about 25 minutes, or until it has become browned and slightly crispy. (Don't cook any longer, otherwise it will come out burnt, even if it doesn't look like it is).

7) Let your granola first cool for about 10 minutes on the baking sheet before cutting it into bars.

8) Transfer granola onto a flat surface and cut it into bar-shapes. Allow it cool off for a bit longer on a wire rack afterwards. Enjoy the highly nutritious, protein-filled cherry quinoa granola either in bar form or crumble as granola pieces (you can use it as a topping for yogurt if you want to mix things up!) Store in an airtight container, and enjoy it for up to 5 days!

(MAKES: 18 bars)

Spanish Breakfast Tortilla

INGREDIENTS:

- 2 small onions, finely diced
- 3 tbsp olive oil
- 10 large eggs
- 1 tsp salt
- 1 tsp ground pepper
- 3 large baking potatoes, peeled and thinly sliced

INSTRUCTIONS:

1)   Place the onions and olive oil in a skillet over medium heat, and slowly cook onions in olive oil until they have become lightly browned and caramelized, for about 5–6 minutes.

2)   Combine eggs, salt and pepper into a large bowl and whisk them together, until smooth.

3)   Layer half of the potatoes and fried onions in a greased 4-quart slow cooker, and follow by placing half of the eggs over the layers. Repeat layers until you've finished pouring in the remainder of the whisked eggs.

4)   Cover and cook on low for 6–7 hours or on high for 3½–4 hours.

SERVES: 6

Vegetable and Egg Scramble with Fontina Cheese

INGREDIENTS:

- 1 tbsp grapeseed oil
- 1 clove garlic, chopped
- 1 cup chopped broccoli
- ½ cup sliced grape tomatoes
- 1 large whole egg
- 2 egg whites
- 2 tbsp fresh basil
- ½ tsp sea salt
- 1 tsp oregano
- 1 tbsp shredded fontina cheese

INSTRUCTIONS:

1) Heat the oil in a medium skillet over medium-high heat. Sauté the garlic for 1 minute, and follow by adding the broccoli and tomatoes, then cook for about

2–3 minutes until broccoli is tender, but is also still crunchy.

2) Whisk your egg and egg whites in a bowl until frothy.

3) Pour egg and egg whites into skillet and continue to mix thoroughly while the eggs cook. Add salt, basil, oregano, and cheese and cook for 3–4 minutes, or until eggs have golden or light brown edges. Remove from heat and serve immediately.

Avocado and Egg Breakfast Burrito

Ingredients:

- 3 large whole eggs
- 3 egg whites
- ¼ cup shredded Cheddar cheese
- 1/3 cup milk
- 1 tbsp grapeseed oil
- ¼ yellow onion, finely chopped
- ½ green pepper, diced
- 2 avocados, peeled, pitted, and mashed
- ¼ tsp salt
- ½ tsp pepper

- 4 gluten-free corn or rice flour tortillas, warmed
- 2/3 cup crumbled goat cheese
- ¼ cup gluten-free salsa

INSTRUCTIONS:

1)   In a medium bowl, beat together the eggs, egg whites, cheese, and milk until the mixture is frothy.

2)   Heat oil in a medium skillet over medium-high heat. Sauté the onion and green pepper until onion has become golden-brown and caramelized, for about 2–3 minutes.

3)   Pour the egg mixture into the skillet and cook while stirring, until eggs are scrambled.

4)   Season the mashed avocados with salt and pepper to taste.

5)   Place tortillas one at a time in a separate skillet and cook until they're warm. This should take about 2–3 minutes.

6)   Spread equal amounts of avocado on one side of each tortilla and layer with equal amounts of goat cheese and scrambled eggs. Roll tortillas up into burritos and serve them immediately (while still warm) with a generous amount of salsa on the side.

The Perfect Lunch Salad

Ingredients:

- 3 celery stalks, very thinly sliced
- 1 cup chickpeas (equivalent 14-ounce can), drained/rinsed
- 3 handfuls arugula or shredded romaine lettuce
- 1/3 cup toasted pepitas or almonds
- 15 black olives, chopped
- 1/2 small red onion, finely diced
- 1 small head of broccoli florets, blanched

Creamy Miso Dressing:

- 1 medium clove garlic, smashed
- 1 tablespoon white miso
- 1 tablespoon mirin
- 1 tablespoon brown rice vinegar
- big pinch of ground cumin
- 1/3 cup / 80 ml plain yogurt
- 1-2 tablespoons heavy cream, or to taste
- 1 small ripe avocado, sliced

Directions:

1) In a large bowl combine the celery, chickpeas, arugula, pepitas, olives, onion, and broccoli. Set aside.

2) Make the salad dressing by smashing the garlic into a paste in a mortar and pestle (you can also use a knife). Stir in the miso, then add the mirin, and vinegar, and mix everything until it is all combined, with a creamy salad dressing consistency. Add the cumin and

the yogurt, and stir again before adding the heavy cream. Taste, and adjust the dressing as desired.

3) Before serving, add half of the dressing to your other ingredients and toss thoroughly. Keep adding more dressing to suit your liking, adding the avocado toward the end so it maintains its structure. Serves 2-4, depending on what else you'll be having on the side. I like to pair the soup with a tuna salad or turkey and cheese sandwich or panini, using gluten free bread.

Grill Marinated Shrimp

Ingredients:

- 1 cup olive oil
- 1/4 cup chopped fresh parsley
- 1 lemon, juiced
- 2 tablespoons hot pepper sauce
- 3 cloves garlic, minced
- 1 tablespoon tomato paste
- 2 teaspoons dried oregano
- 1 teaspoon salt
- 1 teaspoon ground black pepper
- 2 pounds large shrimp, peeled and deveined with tails attached
- Skewers

Directions:

1) In a mixing bowl, mix together parsley, lemon juice, olive oil, hot sauce, tomato paste, oregano, garlic salt, and black pepper. Save a small amount of this mixture for basting later by pouring your leftover marinade into a large resealable plastic bag with the shrimp. Seal the bag and marinate inside of the refrigerator for 2 hours.

2) To cook the dish, preheat your grill to medium-low heat, and follow by threading shrimp onto skewers, piercing once by the tail and once by the head. Then baste your shrimp in the marinade.

3) Lightly oil the grate of your grill, then cook your shrimp for 5 minutes per side (total of 10 minutes), or until the shrimp is pink and opaque. Baste shrimp frequently with prepared marinade.

Stuffed Peppers

Ingredients:

- 1 pound ground beef
- 1/2 cup uncooked long grain white rice
- 1 cup water
- 6 green bell peppers
- 2 (8 ounce) cans tomato sauce
- 1 tablespoon Worcestershire sauce
- 1/4 teaspoon garlic powder

- 1/4 teaspoon onion powder

- salt and pepper to taste
- 1 teaspoon Italian seasoning

Directions:

Preheat oven to 350 degrees F (175 degrees C).

1) Place the rice and water in a saucepan, and bring it to a boil. Reduce heat, then cover your saucepan and cook for approximately 20 minutes. In a skillet over medium heat, cook your beef until it has become evenly browned.

2) Remove and discard the tops, seeds and membranes of your bell peppers. Follow by placing your peppers in a baking dish with the hollowed sides facing upwards. (Slice the bottoms of the peppers if it is necessary so that they will sturdily stand upright).

3) In a bowl, combine and mix together the browned beef, cooked rice, 1 can tomato sauce, Worcestershire sauce, garlic powder, onion powder, salt, and pepper.

4) Spoon an equal amount of the mixture into each individual hollowed pepper. Mix the leftover tomato sauce and Italian seasoning in a bowl, and pour over the mixture over the stuffed peppers.

5) Bake for 1 hour in the preheated oven, and baste with sauce every 15 minutes, until the peppers have gained a tender consistency.

Bacon-wrapped Pork Roast Recipe

Ingredients

- 1 pork loin roast (about 1 1/2 pounds)
- Salt and pepper
- 1 Tbsp olive oil
- 2 Tbsp finely chopped fresh rosemary
- 1/4 lb bacon, thinly sliced
- 1 cup dry white wine

Directions:

1) Sprinkle your roast with salt on all sides, and allow it to sit at room temperature for 1 hour before you intend to roast it.

2) Pre-heat your oven to 375°F (190°C). Follow by patting the pork roast dry with a few paper towels, then sprinkling it with pepper on all sides and with a little more salt. Place one tablespoon of olive oil in a skillet over medium high heat. When the oil is hot and simmering, add the pork roast to the pan and brown it

on each sides (don't flip the roast until it has already browned on one side). This will take approximately 10 minutes. Remove the roast from the pan and transfer it onto a plate.

3)   Rub your pork roast on each side with your minced fresh rosemary. Follow by wrapping the roast in bacon strips. Secure the roast by tying it with some kitchen string to hold the bacon strips in place.

4)   Place your roast in a pan and cook in the oven at 375°F (190°C), occasionally it with the seasoned pan juices, until the internal temperature reaches 145°F (63°C) on a meat thermometer - this will take approximately 35 to 40 minutes. When the roast has reached has finished cooking, remove it from the oven and transfer it onto a serving dish. Cover the roast with foil to keep it warm while you make the pan sauce.

5)   Sauce: Place the roasting pan on top of a stove over low heat. Pour white wine into the pan, and follow by scraping up the browned bits from the bottom of the pan using either a flat edged metal or wood spatula. Then pour your scraped up pan drippings through a fine mesh sieve into a small-sized saucepan. Heat your sauce until it is simmering, then remove sauce from heat and pour into a gravy boat or a bowl. Serve the roast with your freshly made sauce, and enjoy!

Sirloin Steak with Garlic Butter

Ingredients:

- 1/2 cup butter
- 2 teaspoons garlic powder
- 4 cloves of garlic, minced
- 4 pounds beef top sirloin steaks
- Salt and pepper to taste

Directions:

1) Preheat an outdoor grill to high heat.

2) In a small bowl, melt butter mixed with garlic powder and minced garlic, over medium-low heat. Set aside

3) Sprinkle both sides of each steak with salt and pepper.

4) Grill steaks 4 to 5 minutes per side, or to preferred doneness. When finished, transfer to warmed plates. Brush tops liberally with garlic butter and allow to sit for 2 to 3 minutes before serving. Enjoy!

Baked Kale Chips (make a great addition to any lunch!)

Ingredients:

- 1 bag of kale
- 1 tablespoon olive oil
- 1 teaspoon seasoned salt

Directions:

1) Preheat oven to 350 degrees F (175 degrees C). Line a non-insulated cookie sheet with parchment paper.

2) Carefully remove thick stems from the kale with a knife or kitchen shears, and tear into bite-sized pieces. Wash and thoroughly dry kale with a salad spinner. Drizzle kale with olive oil and sprinkle with seasoning salt.

3) Bake for 10-15 minutes until edges are brown but not burnt. Enjoy!

Caramel Apple Pork Chops

Ingredients:

- 4 (3/4 inch) thick pork chops
- 1 teaspoon vegetable oil
- 2 tablespoons brown sugar salt and pepper to taste
- 1/8 teaspoon ground cinnamon
- 1/8 teaspoon ground nutmeg
- 2 tablespoons unsalted butter
- 2 tart apples - peeled, cored and sliced
- 3 tablespoons pecans (optional)

Directions:

1)   Start off by first preheating your oven to 175 degrees F (80 degrees C). Place a medium-sized dish in the oven so it can warm up.

2)   Afterwards, begin cooking the pork chops by first heating a large-sized skillet over medium-high heat. Lightly brush your pork chops with some oil and place into a hot pan. Cook for 5 to 6 minutes (or until finished), while flipping the pork chops occasionally. Transfer to the warm dish, and continue keeping it warm in the preheated oven.

3)   In a small bowl, combine your salt and pepper, brown sugar, cinnamon and nutmeg. Add some butter to the skillet, and follow by stirring in brown sugar mixture and apples. Cover and cook until the apples have become tender. Remove the apples with a slotted spoon and place them on top of your pork chops. Transfer to your preheated oven, to keep the dish warm.

4)   Continue cooking your sauce in an uncovered skillet, until the consistency has slightly thickened. Finally, pour sauce gently over the apples and pork chops. You can sprinkle the dish with chopped pecans if desired.

Black Beans and Quinoa

Ingredients:

- 1 teaspoon vegetable oil

- 1 onion
- chopped 3 cloves garlic
- chopped 3/4 cup quinoa
- 1 1/2 cups vegetable broth

- 1 teaspoon ground cumin
- 1/4 teaspoon cayenne pepper
- salt and ground black pepper to taste
- 1 cup frozen corn kernels
- 2 (15 ounce) cans black beans, rinsed and drained
- 1/2 cup chopped fresh cilantro

Directions:

Heat the oil inside a medium sized saucepan over medium heat, then cook and stir your onion and garlic until they've lightly browned, for about 10 minutes.

Mix your quinoa into the onion mixture and pour over vegetable broth. Follow by seasoning with cumin, cayenne pepper, salt, and pepper. Bring the mixture to a boil. Cover the saucepan, reduce heat, and simmer until quinoa is tender and broth is absorbed, for about 20 minutes.

Stir the frozen corn into the saucepan, and continue to simmer until it has become heated thoroughly, for about 5 minutes. Finally, mix in the black beans and cilantro. Enjoy!

Italian Style Fish Fillets

Ingredients:

2 tablespoons olive oil

1 onion, thinly sliced

2 cloves garlic, minced

1 (14.5 ounce) can diced tomatoes

1/2 cup black olives, pitted and sliced

1 tablespoon chopped fresh parsley

1/2 cup dry white wine

1 pound cod fillets

Directions:

1)   In a large frying pan, heat the oil over medium heat, then sauté your onions and garlic in olive oil until they have become softened. Stir in your tomatoes, parsley, olives, and wine, and let simmer for 5 minutes.

2)   Place fillets in sauce. Simmer for approximately 5 more minutes, or until fish turns white and is fully cooled. Enjoy!

Juicy Seasoned Roasted Chicken

Ingredients:

- 1 (3 pound) whole chicken giblets removed
- salt and black pepper to taste
- 1 tablespoon onion powder
- 1/2 cup margarine
- divided 1 stalk celery, leaves removed

Directions:

1) Preheat oven to 350 degrees F (175 degrees C).

2) Place chicken into a roasting pan, and season the chicken generously on each side with salt and pepper. Sprinkle each side with onion powder as well. Place 3 tablespoons of margarine (you can also use butter) into the middle of chicken cavity. Place dollops of the remaining margarine (or butter) around all sides of the chicken's exterior. Finally, chop the celery into 3 or 4 pieces, and then place it into the chicken cavity.

3) Bake uncovered for approximately 1 hour and 15 minutes in the preheated oven at a minimum internal temperature of 180 degrees F (82 degrees C). Remove the chicken from heat, and baste it with the melted butter or margarine and drippings. Proceed by covering your chicken with aluminum foil, and allow it sit for about 30 minutes before serving.

Shrimp and Cheddar Grits

Ingredients

- 1 14-ounce can reduced-sodium chicken broth
- 1 1/2 cups water
- 3/4 cup quick grits, (not instant) (see Shopping Tip)
- 1/2 teaspoon freshly ground pepper, divided
- 3/4 cup extra-sharp or sharp Cheddar cheese
- 1 pound peeled and deveined raw shrimp, (16-20 per pound; see Shopping Tip)
- 1 bunch scallions, trimmed and cut into 1-inch pieces
- 1 tablespoon extra-virgin olive oil
- 1/4 teaspoon garlic powder
- 1/8 teaspoon salt

Directions:

1) Position rack in upper third of oven; preheat broiler.

2) Bring broth and water to a boil in a large saucepan over medium-high heat. Whisk in grits and 1/4 teaspoon pepper. Reduce heat to medium-low, cover and cook, stirring occasionally, until thickened, 5 to 7

minutes. Remove from heat and stir in cheese. Cover to keep warm.

3) Meanwhile, toss shrimp, oil, scallions garlic powder, the leftover 1/4 teaspoon of pepper and salt (to taste) into a medium to large sized bowl. Transfer to a baking sheet. Broil the shrimp and stir them once, until the shrimp are pink and opaque and appropriately cooked, for approximately 5 to 6 minutes. Serve the grits along with the broiled shrimp and scallions. Enjoy!

Baked Shrimp in Tomato Feta Sauce Recipe

Ingredients:

- 1 Tbsp olive oil
- 1 medium onion, chopped
- 2 cloves garlic, minced
- 2 14.5-ounce cans of diced tomatoes
- 1/4 cup minced fresh parsley
- 1 Tbsp minced fresh dill or 1 teaspoon dried dill
- 1 to 1 1/4 pounds medium sized raw shrimp, peeled and deveined (can leave tails on), thaw if frozen
- Pinch of salt, more to taste
- Pinch black pepper, more to taste
- 3 ounces feta cheese (about 2/3 cup, crumbled)

Directions:

1) Preheat oven to 425°F. Heat your oil in a large, oven-proof skillet on medium high heat. Add the onions and cook until they're softened, for 3-5 minutes. Add the garlic and cook until it's noticeably fragrant, about 30 seconds more.

2) Add the tomatoes and bring to a simmer, and then reduce the heat and let simmer for 5-10 minutes, or until the juices have thickened a bit.

3) Remove from heat. Add in the herbs, shrimp, feta cheese, and salt and pepper to taste, and stir it around to mix well. Place pan in oven and bake, with the pan uncovered, until shrimp are cooked through - this will take about 10-12 minutes.

Serve immediately over rice.

Brown Butter Harvest Cake with Vanilla Nut Cream

Ingredients:

For the Harvest Cake:

- 2 sticks (225 g) unsalted butter
- 3-1/2 cups (400 g) blanched almond flour

- ½ cup coconut flour (60 g) coconut flour
- 2 teaspoon (7 g) baking powder
- ¾ teaspoon (3 g) sea salt
- 2 teaspoons (7s g) cinnamon
- 1 teaspoon (4 g) nutmeg
- ¾ cup (165 g) raw honey
- 2 teaspoons (6 g) vanilla extract
- 4 large eggs
- 1 cup (235 ml / 8 oz) unsweetened coconut milk
- ¾ cup (175 ml / 6 oz) fresh pressed apple cider or juice
- 1 cup (130 g) grated carrot
- 1 cup (130 g) grated zucchini

For the Nutty Vanilla Creme:

- 1-1/2 cups raw cashews, soaked
- ¾ cup fresh apple cider or juice
- 3 Medjool dates, pit removed
- 1-1/2 tablespoons raw honey
- 1 vanilla bean, seeds scraped
- (Optional: fresh flowers for decorating)

Directions:

1) To make the cake, start with making the brown butter first. Place butter in a small to medium saucepan over medium heat and melt it until it has become

golden brown or dark amber - this should take 8 to 10 minutes.

2)   Preheat the oven to 350 F (180 C). In the meantime, grease two 6-inch round cake pans. Line the bottom of cake pans with parchment paper.

3)   In the bowl of an electric mixer fitted with a paddle, combine all of the dry ingredients: almond and coconut flours, baking powder, salt, cinnamon, and nutmeg. Mix together these ingredients on low speed for 1 to 2 minutes.

4)   In a separate bowl, whisk together your honey, butter, vanilla extract, eggs, coconut milk, and apple cider or juice.

5)   Pour the wet ingredients (honey, butter, vanilla extract, eggs, coconut milk, apple cider/juice) onto the dry ingredients and mix everything on medium-low speed. You can also mix this by hand if you don't have access to electric mixer.

6)   Fold in grated carrot and zucchini.

7)   Pour the batter in the cake pans and cook 35 to 40 minutes, or until a tester inserted comes out clean.

8)   To make the nutty vanilla creme "icing", combine all the ingredients in a blender or a food processor.

9)   Blend until smooth.

10) After the cakes are done baking, let them cool in the pans for 15 minutes.

11) Turn over to a cooling rack and carefully remove parchment paper, letting it sit for another 20 minutes or until the cakes have cooled.

12) When cakes are cool enough, place the bottom layer of the cake on a plate or a stand, with the flat bottom facing upwards.

13) Spread the vanilla creme on the cake with an offset spatula. This will be your cake's middle filling.

14) Gently place the second cake on top of the bottom layer, and spread more vanilla creme on the cake's surface.

Optional: You can decorate the cake with fresh flowers.

To make the crust.

1) Combine millet flour, almond flour and salt in a food processor.

2) Heat coconut oil and maple syrup over low heat, then stir to combine.

3) Add your coconut oil and maple syrup to the flour and pulse thoroughly until well-mixed.

4) Spread out the dough in a 9.5 inch oiled tart pan (preferably with a removable bottom), press down and fill sides to form a crust.

5) Pierce the crust with a fork several times, then bake for 15 minutes.

6) Remove the crust from oven and flatten it with a fork, pressing down to make it as compact as possible

For the filling:

1)   Peel 4 apples, slice them thinly and pile into pan.

2)   Mix together your maple syrup and lemon juice and brush the mixture over the apples.

3)   Sprinkle over the almonds and bake for 1 hour (this could take a little more or less longer, depending on your oven) until the apples have become soft and slightly browned

Glaze:

1)   Mix together apricot jam and water in a small pan and place over low heat until the preserves are thinned.

2)   Remove the mixture from heat and add lemon juice, then put it through a strainer to remove any apricot chunks, if necessary.

3)   Brush the tart with your glaze and serve warm. Enjoy!

Raspberry Lemon Cheesecake Bites

Ingredients:

- 1 tablespoon flax seed, freshly ground
- 2 tablespoons warm water
- 1/3 cup coconut oil
- 1/3 cup dairy free cream cheese (non hydrogenated), softened

- 1/2 cup sugar (agave, coconut nectar, raw sugar)
- 1 cup gluten free all purpose flour
- 1 teaspoon baking powder
- 1/2 teaspoon xanthan gum
- pinch salt
- 3/4 pint fresh raspberries
- zest of 1/2 small lemon

Directions:

1) Preheat oven to 350 degrees.

2) Grind flax seeds in either a blender or a coffee grinder – both work well. Place 1 tablespoon of ground flax in a bowl, add the water and stir. Place in refrigerator to form into a gel (this equals/replaces one egg).

3) Mix together coconut oil, cream cheese, and sugar, forming it into a cream texture, and then stir in your flax mixture. Add flour onto the top of this mixture, but do not stir. Add baking powder, xanthan gum and salt, and stir it into the flour before combining flour with coconut cream cheese. Then fold in your raspberries and lemon zest. Drop cookies by the spoonful onto prepared baking sheet, and bake at 350 degrees F for approximately 15 minutes. Let cool and enjoy!

Gluten-Free Garbanzo Bean Chocolate Cake

Ingredients:

- 1 1/2 cups semisweet chocolate chips
- 1 (19 ounce) can of garbanzo beans, rinsed and drained
- 4 eggs
- 3/4 cup white sugar
- 1/2 teaspoon baking powder
- 1 tablespoon confectioners' sugar for dusting

Directions:

1)   Preheat oven to 350 degrees F (175 degrees C). Grease a 9 inch round cake pan.

2)   Place the chocolate chips into a microwave-safe bowl. Cook in the microwave for about 2 minutes, stirring every 20 seconds after first minute of cooking, until chocolate is melted and smooth.

3)   Combine the beans and eggs in the bowl of a food processor. Process until smooth. Add the sugar and baking power and pulse to blend. Pour in the melted chocolate and blend until smooth, scraping down the corners to make sure chocolate is completely mixed. Pour the batter into the prepared cake pan.

4)   Bake in preheated oven for 40 minutes, or until a knife or toothpick is inserted in the middle of the cake and comes out clean. Cool in the pan on a wire rack for 10 to 15 minutes before placing onto a serving plate. Dust with confectioners' sugar right before serving. Enjoy!

Gluten-Free Chocolate Chip Cookies

Ingredients:

- 3/4 cup butter, softened
- 1 1/4 cups packed brown sugar
- 1/4 cup white sugar
- 1 teaspoon gluten-free vanilla extract
- 1/4 cup egg substitute
- 2 1/4 cups gluten-free baking mix
- 1 teaspoon baking soda
- 1 teaspoon baking powder
- 1 teaspoon salt
- 12 ounces semisweet chocolate chips

Directions:

1)   Preheat oven to 375 degrees F (190 degrees C). Prepare a greased baking sheet.

2)   In a medium bowl, cream butter and sugar. Gradually add egg substitute and vanilla extract while mixing. Sift together gluten-free flour mix, baking soda, baking powder and salt. Stir into butter mixture until blended. Finally, stir in the chocolate chips.

3)   Using a teaspoon, drop cookies 2 inches apart onto prepared baking sheet. Bake in preheated oven for 6 to 8 minutes or until light brown. Let cookies cool on baking sheet for 2 minutes before placing on wire racks. Enjoy!

Strawberry Soup

- 2 cups frozen strawberries
- 2 cups milk 1 cup heavy cream
- 1/2 cup sour cream
- 2 tablespoons white sugar, or to taste

Directions:

Blend your strawberries, milk, cream and sour cream in a blender or food processor until smooth, then stir in sugar to taste. Chill for 8 hours or overnight in the refrigerator before serving. Enjoy!

Chocolate Pudding Cups

Ingredients:

- 2/3 cup granulated sugar
- 2 tablespoons cornstarch
- 1/8 teaspoon kosher salt
- 3 cups whole milk
- 4 large egg yolks
- 1/2 teaspoon pure vanilla extract
- 6 ounces bittersweet chocolate chopped
- 1/2 teaspoon unsweetened cocoa powder

Directions:

1) Start by combining the sugar, cornstarch, and salt in a medium saucepan. Add 1/3 cup of the milk, and stir it in until a smooth paste has formed. Whisk in the egg yolks and the remainder of your milk.

2) Cook the mixture over medium-low heat, and stir it constantly with a wooden spoon or a spatula until it has thickened, for about 12 to 15 minutes (do not allow to boil). Remove from heat.

3) Add the vanilla and chocolate to the mixture, and stir until the chocolate is melted and the mixture is smooth. Follow by pouring the pudding into eight 4-ounce ramekins, glasses, or teacups. Refrigerate, covered, until chilled, for a minimum of 2 hours and up to 2 days. Sprinkle with the cocoa powder before serving, and enjoy!

Peach and Raspberry Parfait

Ingredients:

- 2 peaches, cut into 2 1/2-inch pieces
- 1 1/2 cups raspberries
- 2 tablespoons sugar
- 1 tablespoon fresh lemon juice
- 1 pint vanilla ice cream

Directions:

1) Combine your raspberries, sugar, peaches and lemon juice and place them into a large sized bowl. Allow them to sit for 20 minutes, tossing once.

2) Place scoops of ice cream into bowls or glasses. Finally, top the ice cream with the fruit mixture, transforming it into a delicious raspberry-peach parfait. Enjoy!

Conclusion

Now that you are well-informed about all of the essential key facts about gluten, you can implement this useful, important information into your lifestyle, whether you have coeliac disease, gluten-sensitivity or are simply looking for ways to improve the health benefits of your palate for reasons such as weight-loss and increased energy levels.

A gluten-free diet will eliminate a number of unnecessary, fattening gluten-based starchy foods and will replace them with healthier, well-balanced quality foods like lean proteins and plenty of antioxidant-filled, healthy vegetables and fruits, which significantly contribute to overall improved health. It will also provide relief to a wide array of health concerns and gluten-intolerance symptoms in those suffering from coeliac disease and gluten-sensitivity.

Overall, a gluten-free diet holds a wide array of benefits and holds the potential to significantly improve your health and well-being, which in turn will lead to a better quality of life. Your body will certainly thank you!

Part 2

Introduction

Congratulations on taking your first step towards being healthy! As you might know, people with the Celiac diseases and/or allergies need to adhere to a gluten free diet in order to enjoy a normal life. Gluten is a type of protein that is usually found in foods such as wheat or barley, and in some regions, these grains are the staple diet for their population. A gluten diet may also be referred to as a wheat free diet. The good news is there are many substitutes available in the market that are gluten free and also help you diversify your meal options. Rice, millet and quinoa are the popular substitutes for barley or even wheat-based meals.

Gluten free diet is not only meant for those with the disease or the allergies, but it can also for those who want to maintain a healthy diet and incorporate a lot of protein and carbohydrates in to their diet. Usually, Gluten is the protein that is found in wheat, which gives the elasticity to dough and helps it maintain its shape and rise. Gluten is also a complex combination of two proteins known as Gliadin and Glutenin that are joined by starch components and is found in various grains. While Glutenin is the major type of protein found in wheat flour, Gliadin is responsible for the bread to rise properly and this makes for about 47% of the total protein content in the grain.

While you may assume that only those with the Celiac Disease are the ones intolerant to Gluten, it is found that in many cases, you might simply have intolerance to Gluten. It might just be an autoimmune reaction that your body may have, since the immune system does not recognize these particles entering the body and might attack it for protection. Anybody who is intolerant to Gluten might face an immediate reaction right after the consumption of foods containing gluten. They might experience some bloating of tissues, diarrhea, abdominal cramping and even flatulence.

While being on a Gluten free diet is essential for those with the Celiac Disease or allergies, it is important to know that not all of us need to maintain such a diet. But this diet offers a variety of health benefits by helping you eliminate foods from your unhealthy diet such as processed foods, fast foods, fried foods, etc. It also helps in improving cholesterol levels, increasing energy levels and promotes digestive health. While you are working on your health you can shed a couple of pounds too!

This book contains gluten free recipes that can help you and your family to lead a healthy lifestyle and a tasty one too!

So read on!

Chapter 1: Gluten free Breads

Almond Buns

Ingredients:

- 1 ½ cups almond flour
- 4 large eggs, whisked
- 10 tablespoons unsalted butter, melted
- 3 teaspoons splenda (optional)
- 3 teaspoons baking powder

Method:

1. Mix together flour, splenda, and baking powder in a large bowl.
2. Add eggs and whisk. Add butter and continue whisking.
3. Grease muffin molds.
4. Pour into muffin molds (only half fill the molds).
5. Bake in a preheated oven at 350 degree F for about 15-17 minutes or until done.
6. Cool on a wire rack.

Garlic Dill Dinner Rolls

Ingredients:

- 5 cups gluten free all-purpose baking flour
- 3 cups warm water (110 degree F)
- 4 teaspoons xanthan gum
- 2 tablespoons white sugar
- 2 teaspoons salt
- 2 packages (0.25 ounce each) rapid rise yeast
- 4 teaspoons dried dill
- 6 large eggs
- 3 teaspoons garlic, minced
- 3 teaspoons canola oil
- 2 teaspoons apple cider vinegar

Method:

1. Add warm water to a bowl. Add sugar and stir until dissolved.
2. Sprinkle yeast over the water and leave it aside for 5 minutes. It would have begun to foam.
3. Whisk together eggs, oil and vinegar in another bowl. Whisk until nice and frothy.
4. Add flour, xanthan gum and salt to a large bowl and mix until well combined.
5. Gently pour the warm water mixture into the flour mixture using an electric mixture with a dough attachment or add it to the food processor with a dough attachment.
6. Gently add the egg mixture and beat until it is just mixed. Add dill and garlic. Beat the dough for about

4 minutes on high speed until the dough is held together.
7. Cover the bowl with a cling wrap and keep it in a warm place for at least 30 minutes.
8. Grease 2 baking sheets or baking dishes.
9. Shape into 24 large rolls and place on the baking dish. Give a gap of at least an inch between 2 rolls.
10. Bake in a preheated oven in batches at 350 degree F until they are light golden in color.

French bread (baguette)

Ingredients:

- 2 cups tapioca flour
- 2 cups brown rice flour
- 2 cups sorghum flour
- 4 tablespoons active dry yeast
- 4 teaspoons xanthan gum
- 3 teaspoons salt
- 2 cups warm water (110 degree F)
- 2 teaspoons apple cider vinegar
- 2 tablespoons olive oil
- 6 egg whites or 2 whole eggs and 4 egg whites

Method:

1. Add warm water to a bowl. Add sugar and stir until dissolved.
2. Sprinkle yeast over the water and leave it aside for 5 minutes. It would have begun to foam.

3. Whisk together eggs, oil and vinegar in another bowl. Whisk until nice and frothy.
4. Mix all the flours together.
5. Add flour mixture, xanthan gum and salt to a large bowl and mix until well combined.
6. Gently pour the warm water mixture into the flour mixture using an electric mixture with a dough attachment or add it to the food processor with a dough attachment.
7. Gently add the egg mixture and beat until it is just mixed. Beat the dough for about 4 minutes on high speed until the dough is held together.
8. Grease 2 baking sheets.
9. Divide and shape the dough into 4 baguettes. Place 2 baguettes on each of the baking sheet. Make 3 cuts on each of the baguettes with a sharp knife.
10. Keep aside for at least 30 minutes to rise.
11. Brush the top of the baguettes lightly with olive oil.
12. Bake in a preheated oven at 400 degree F for about 30 minutes or until done.
13. It tastes best the day it is baked. Unused ones can be wrapped in aluminum foil and store.

Sandwich Bread

Ingredients:

- 1/2 cup sorghum flour
- 2 tablespoons whole flax meal
- 14 tablespoons gluten free all-purpose baking flour or brown rice flour blend
- 1/2 teaspoon xanthan gum
- 1 teaspoon instant yeast
- 1/2 teaspoon salt
- 1/2 cup milk at room temperature
- 2 small eggs
- 1 tablespoon vegetable oil or melted butter
- 1 tablespoon molasses
- 3/4 teaspoon baking powder

Method:

1. Mix together flax meal, flours, yeasts, baking powder, salt and xanthan gum.
2. Whisk together eggs, oil or butter, milk, and molasses in another bowl. Whisk until nice and frothy.
3. Add the flour mixture into the milk mixture. Add 1/2 cup at a time and beat each time. Continue until all the dry ingredients and well blended into the milk mixture to form a thick, smooth batter.

4. Cover the bowl and keep it aside for at least an hour to rise.
5. Scrape the sides and beat the batter for a minute.
6. Pour into a greased loaf pan. Cover loosely with a cling wrap and keep aside for about 1 1/2 to 2 hours for the batter to rise.
7. Bake in a preheated oven at 350 degree F for about 40 minutes or until done. An instant read thermometer when inserted in the center should show a reading of 205 degree F when the loaf is fully baked.
8. Remove the loaf pan from the oven. Loosen the sides and remove the bread and place on a wire rack to cool.
9. Slice when it cools completely and serve.

Zucchini Bread

Ingredients:

- 1 cup coconut flour
- 1 ½ teaspoon baking soda
- 1 teaspoon salt
- 2 tablespoons ground cinnamon
- ½ teaspoon nutmeg
- 8 eggs
- 1 ½ tablespoons raw honey
- 2 cups zucchini, finely shredded, squeezed of all the moisture
- 2 ripe bananas, mashed

- 2 tablespoons coconut oil
- 1 cup walnuts, chopped, (optional)

Method:

1. Add eggs, honey, oil, and banana to a bowl and mix well.
2. Add zucchini, coconut flour, baking soda, salt, cinnamon and nutmeg. Mix well until you get a smooth batter. Add walnuts and stir.
3. Pour the batter into a greased bread pan (fill it ¾ full). Bake in a preheated oven at 350 degree F for about 45 minutes or until done.
4. Remove from oven and place on wire rack to cool for a while
5. Run a knife along the sides to loosen the edges. Invert on to a plate.
6. When cooled completely, slice and serve.

Chapter 2: Gluten free Dips Recipes

Roasted Sweet Onion Dip

Ingredients:

- 4 large Vidalia or any other variety of sweet onions, peeled, quartered
- 2 whole garlic heads
- 2 tablespoons olive oil
- 2/3 cup low fat sour cream
- 2 teaspoons salt, divided
- 1/2 cup fresh parsley, chopped
- 2 tablespoons fresh lemon juice

Method:

1. Discard the outer white thin skin from the garlic heads (do not separate into cloves of garlic and do not peel it either. The garlic should remain whole).
2. Wrap the garlic in aluminum foil.
3. Add onions to a bowl and sprinkle oil over it. Season with salt. Toss well.
4. Place onion and wrapped garlic on a baking sheet and bake in a preheated oven at 425 degree F for an hour.
5. Remove from the oven and cool for a while. Chop the onions finely. Now separate the garlic cloves

and extract the pulp of garlic by squeezing. Discard the skin of the garlic.
6. Mix together onion, garlic and rest of the ingredients in a bowl. Cover and refrigerate for at least an hour.

Hummus

Ingredients:

- 2 cans chickpeas (garbanzo beans), rinsed, drained
- 1 lemon, juiced
- 2 cloves garlic, minced
- ½ cup tahini or more to suit your taste
- 6 tablespoons olive oil
- 6 tablespoons water, plus more if needed
- 1 teaspoon cumin
- Salt to taste
- Pepper powder, to taste
- Smoked paprika to taste (optional)

Method:

1. Blend together all the ingredients until smooth.
2. Serve

Healthy Broccoli Guacamole:

Ingredients:

- 4 ripe avocados, peeled, diced
- 1 ½ cups broccoli florets, minced
- 2 tomatoes, diced
- ½ cup red onions, finely chopped
- 2 cloves garlic, minced
- 2 tablespoons lemon juice
- 2 tablespoons fresh cilantro, chopped
- Salt to taste

Method:

1. Mix together all the ingredients and serve.

Tomato salsa

Ingredients:

- 4 medium tomatoes, deseeded, finely chopped
- ¼ cup green onion, minced
- ¼ cup fresh cilantro
- 1 small green bell pepper, finely chopped
- 1 teaspoon chili flakes or cayenne pepper
- 3 tablespoons lime juice
- 4 tablespoons extra virgin olive oil
- 1 teaspoon sea salt

Method:

1. Mix together all the ingredients in a bowl.

Creamy Curry Cashew Dip

Ingredients:

- 1/2 cup raw cashew
- 1 1/2 tablespoons lemon juice
- 6 tablespoons mayonnaise
- 3 tablespoons coconut milk
- Zest of half a lemon, grated
- 1/8 teaspoon garlic powder
- 1/4 teaspoon curry powder
- A pinch cayenne pepper
- A pinch salt or to taste
- 1 tablespoon honey or to taste
- Freshly ground black pepper to taste

Method:

1. Add cashews and mayonnaise to a blender and blend until smooth. Add coconut milk and blend again.
2. Add rest of the ingredients and blend again.
3. Taste and adjust the seasoning if necessary.
4. Chill in the refrigerator before use.

Baba Ghanoush

Ingredients:

- 1 large eggplant
- 1 tablespoon tahini
- 1 clove garlic, minced
- 1 1/2 teaspoons extra virgin olive oil
- 1 tablespoon fresh lemon juice
- 1/2 teaspoon cumin powder (optional)
- Salt to taste
- Pepper powder to taste
- 2 tablespoons fresh parsley for garnishing

Method:

1. Roast the eggplant either in an oven at 400 degree F or grill it.
2. Place the roasted eggplant in a bowl of cold water and let it remain in it for a while. Remove the skin and discard it.
3. Place the eggplant along with rest of ingredients except parsley in a blender and blend until smooth.
4. Transfer into a bowl and refrigerate until use.
5. Before serving drizzle some more olive oil on top. Sprinkle parsley and serve.

Chapter 3: Gluten free Smoothie Recipes

Apple Pie Green Smoothie:

Ingredients:

- 2 cups water
- 1 cup apple juice, unsweetened
- 2 tablespoons walnuts, chopped
- 1 teaspoon ground cinnamon or to taste
- ½ teaspoon vanilla extract or maple extract
- A large pinch ground nutmeg
- 1 English cucumber, chopped
- 4 cups spinach
- 2 apples, cored, chopped
- ½ avocado, peeled, pitted, chopped, frozen

Method:

1. Blend together all the ingredients of the smoothie until smooth. Add more water if the smoothie is too thick.
2. Serve in tall glasses with crushed ice.

Cranberry & raspberry smoothie

Ingredients:

- 1 1/2 cups cranberry juice
- 1 cup milk of your choice
- 1 1/2 cups frozen raspberries
- 3-4 drops stevia or to taste or any sweetener of your choice
- A few mint leaves

Method:

1. Blend together all the ingredients of the smoothie except mint until smooth. Add more water if the smoothie is too thick.
2. Serve in tall glasses with crushed ice.

Mango, Lime n Jalapeno Smoothie:

Ingredients:

- 2 small bananas, peeled, sliced
- 1 ½ cups frozen mango
- 1 small jalapeno pepper, chopped
- 1 cup unsweetened almond milk or coconut milk
- 2 tablespoons flaxseed, ground
- 2 tablespoons chia seeds, ground
- 4 tablespoons hemp seed, ground
- 1 lime, freshly squeezed
- 1 avocado (optional)

Method:

1. Blend together all the ingredients of the smoothie until smooth. Add more milk if the smoothie is too thick.
2. Serve in tall glasses with ice.

Energy Boosting Smoothie

Ingredients:

- 2 bananas, peeled and sliced
- 16 ounces Greek yogurt
- 4 tablespoons peanut butter
- 4 tablespoons cocoa powder
- 1/2 teaspoon ground cinnamon
- Ice cubes as required

Method:

1. Add all the ingredients to the blender and blend until smooth. Add yogurt or water to dilute the smoothie if you desire a smoothie of thinner consistency.
2. Pour into tall glasses and serve.

Flat - Belly Smoothie

Ingredients:

- 1 cup frozen blueberries
- 1 cup frozen pineapple, chopped
- 2 cups kale, hard stems and ribs removed, torn
- 6 ounces vanilla flavored, nonfat Greek yogurt
- 1 1/2 cups water

Method:

1. Add all the ingredients to the blender and blend until smooth. Add more water to dilute the smoothie if you desire a smoothie of thinner consistency.
2. Pour into tall glasses.
3. Serve with crushed ice.

Blueberry Tofu Protein Smoothie:

Ingredients:

- 1 cup blueberries
- 2 tablespoons honey or to taste
- 1 large banana, peeled and sliced
- 8 ounces soft silken tofu
- 2 cups soy milk or more according to the consistency you desire

Method:

1. Add all the ingredients to the blender and blend until smooth. Add more soymilk to dilute the smoothie if you desire a smoothie of thinner consistency.
2. Pour into tall glasses and serve with crushed ice.

Chapter 4: Gluten free Breakfast Recipes

All in one Baked Mushrooms

Ingredients:

- 6 eggs
- 6 large mushrooms
- 3 tablespoons olive oil
- 6 slices ham
- Baked beans to serve

Method:

1. Place mushrooms in a greased baking dish. Sprinkle oil all over the mushrooms.
2. Place the dish in a preheated oven at 430 degree F for 15 minutes or until soft.
3. Remove the dish from the oven. Wrap a ham slice over each mushroom to make pockets.
4. Break an egg into each of the pockets. Place the dish back into the oven and bake for around 10 minutes or until the whites are set.
5. Serve with baked beans.

Smoked Salmon Frittata:

Ingredients:

- ½ lb new potatoes, cut into thick slices
- 0.22 lbs smoked salmon, cut into wide strips
- 4 large eggs, whisked well
- 1 tablespoon dill, chopped
- ½ cup frozen green peas
    - Cooking spray

Method:

1. Par boil the potato slices in salt water. Drain and keep aside to cool.
2. Add salmon to the beaten eggs. Also add dill, green peas, salt, and pepper. Mix well.
3. Add the potatoes.
4. Spray a nonstick frying pan with olive oil. Place the pan over low heat. Pour the egg mixture into the pan. Cook for about 12-15 minutes until the eggs have set.
5. Gently flip sides and cook the other side too.
6. Cut into wedges and serve.

Rice and Raisin Breakfast Pudding:

Ingredients:

- ½ cup water
- 1 ½ cups cooked brown rice
- ¼ cup raisins
- 2 tablespoons maple syrup
- ½ cup soy milk
- ¼ cup almonds, chopped, toasted
- ½ teaspoon ground cinnamon
- ¼ teaspoon ground cardamom

Method:

1. To a thick-bottomed saucepan add all the ingredients. Place the saucepan over medium heat. Bring to a boil.
2. Lower the heat and simmer for 6-8 minutes until it thickens. Stir in between a couple of times.
3. Serve in individual bowls.

Quinoa Porridge:

Ingredients:

- 1 cup quinoa
- ½ teaspoon ground cinnamon
- 3 cups almond milk
- 1 cup water
- ¼ cup brown sugar
- 1 teaspoon vanilla extract (optional)
- A large pinch salt

Method:

1. Place a thick-bottomed saucepan over medium heat. Add quinoa and roast for a couple of minutes until the quinoa is lightly toasted. Add cinnamon and sauté for a few seconds.
2. Add almond milk, water, vanilla, salt, and brown sugar. Mix well.
3. Bring to a boil. Stir frequently.
4. Lower heat and simmer for about 30 minutes until the quinoa is cooked. If it is too, thick, add some more water or almond milk.
5. Serve hot or warm.

Potato & Paprika Tortilla

Ingredients:

- 1 pound new potatoes, rinsed, thickly sliced
- 3 tablespoons olive oil
- 4 cloves garlic, chopped
- 1 large onion, halved, sliced
- 12 eggs
- 1 teaspoon dried oregano
- 1 teaspoon smoked paprika
- ½ cup parsley, chopped + extra for garnishing
- Salt to taste
- Pepper powder to taste

Method:

1. Place a nonstick frying pan over medium heat. Add oil. When oil is heated, add potatoes, onion and garlic and cook until the potatoes are tender. Add paprika and fry for a few seconds.
2. Meanwhile beat eggs along with oregano, salt, pepper, and parsley.
3. Lower heat to minimum. Pour the egg mixture into the pan of potatoes. Mix well until the egg is well coated with the potatoes. Now do not stir anymore and let it cook until the bottom side is golden brown. Flip sides and cook the other side too.
4. Garnish with parsley and serve warm.

Chickpea Pancakes:

Ingredients:

- 2 cups chickpea flour
- 2 cups canned cannellini beans or white kidney beans, drained, rinsed
- 1 tablespoon cilantro, chopped
- Salt and pepper to taste
- 1 teaspoon garlic, minced

Method:

1. Whisk together chickpea flour, 2 ½ cups water, salt, and pepper in a large bowl. Keep aside for an hour.
2. Place a nonstick pan over medium heat. Spray with cooking spray. Make pancakes with the batter. When the bottom side is cooked, flip sides and cook the other side too. Either make small pancakes or make a large one and cut into wedges.
3. Blend together the remaining ingredients until smooth. Add salt and pepper to taste.
4. Spread the pureed beans on the pancakes and serve.

Chapter 5: Gluten free Salad Recipes

The Big Salad:

Ingredients:

- 2 large sweet potatoes, sliced into 1cm thick rounds
- 1 cup toasted sliced almonds
- 2 head romaine, chopped, washed, dried
- 1 red pepper, chopped
- 1 yellow pepper, chopped
- 2 large carrots, julienned
- 1 cucumber, diced
- 4 green onions, thinly sliced
- ¼ cup cilantro or parsley, chopped
- 1 tablespoon coconut oil or grape seed oil

For the dressing:

- 2 cloves garlic, minced
- ½ cup raw almond butter (or roasted peanut butter)
- ¼ cup fresh lime juice
- 4 tablespoons low-sodium tamari
- ¼ cup water
- 2 teaspoons maple syrup or to taste
- 2 teaspoons toasted sesame oil, to taste (optional)
- 2 teaspoons freshly grated ginger (optional)

Method:

1. Brush the sweet potato rounds with oil. Place on a lined baking sheet. Sprinkle salt and pepper.

2. Bake in a preheated oven at 400 degree F for about 30 minutes or until cooked.
3. Flip sides in between. Cook the other side too. To serve, remove from oven
4. To make the dressing: Blend together all the ingredients of the dressing until smooth. Keep aside until use.
5. To assemble the salad. Take a large bowl. Add lettuce. Next layer the vegetables, as you desire. Layer the almonds too. Chill in the refrigerator until use.
6. To serve, add the dressing. Toss and serve.

Edamame Salad:

Ingredients:

- ½ pound frozen edamame, shelled, prepared according to the instructions on the package
- 1 ½ cups frozen corn kernels
- ½ red bell pepper, chopped
- ½ cup green onions, sliced
- ¼ cup red onions, finely chopped
- ½ cup fresh Italian parsley, chopped
- 1 tablespoon fresh oregano or marjoram or basil, chopped

For the dressing:

- ¼ cup fresh lemon juice
- 1 tablespoon Dijon mustard
- 1 tablespoon olive oil
- ½ teaspoon salt
- ½ teaspoon freshly ground black pepper to taste

Method:

1. Mix together all the ingredients of the dressing and keep aside until use.
2. Mix together all the ingredients of the salad. Pour dressing on top. Toss and serve.

Grapefruit, Agave & Pistachio salad

Ingredients:

- 2 white grapefruits, peeled, deseeded, separate into segments, remove the inner skin too
- 2 pink grapefruits
- 1 tablespoon pistachio nuts, chopped
- 2 tablespoons agave nectar
- Pepper powder to taste
- Salt to taste

Method:

1. Place the grapefruits in a large bowl. Add salt and pepper to taste.
2. Sprinkle salt, pepper and pistachio nuts

Spicy Slaw

Ingredients:

- 1 head purple cabbage, shredded
- 2 carrots, peeled, grated
- 2 jalapeno peppers, deseeded, minced
- 2 bunches cilantro, finely chopped

For dressing:

- ¼ cup lime juice
- ¼ cup olive oil
- 2 teaspoon ginger, minced
- 10-15 drops stevia
- 1 teaspoon Celtic sea salt`

Method:

1. Add all the ingredients of the dressing to a small bowl and whisk well.
2. Add rest of the salad ingredients to a bowl. Pour the dressing and toss well.

Chapter 6: Gluten free Snacks Recipes

Cauliflower Tostadas:

Ingredients:

- 12 ounce bag cauliflower, grated, cooked
- 2 eggs
- 2 cups cheese
- Salt and pepper to taste

Method:

1. Mix together all the ingredients.
2. Grease a cookie sheet. Make around 5 inch diameter circles with the mixture on the cookie sheet.
3. Bake in a preheated oven at 450 degree F for about 10-12 minutes.
4. Flip the circles and bake for 5-7 minutes more.
5. Let it cool on a wire rack.
6. Serve with a filling of your choice or have it as it is.

Zucchini Pizza bites:

Ingredients:

- 1 large zucchini, cut into thick slices
- 1 cup pizza sauce
- 1 cup low fat mozzarella cheese, grated
- Pizza toppings of your choice
- 2 tablespoons Italian seasoning

Method:

1. Preheat a grill.
2. Brush both sides of the zucchini slices with olive oil.
3. Grill the zucchini slices for about 8-10 minutes until the zucchini is slightly getting to be tender.
4. Spread pizza sauce over the grilled zucchini slices. Sprinkle topping. Top with cheese.
5. Grill until the cheese is light golden brown.
6. Serve hot.

Puffed Quinoa Peanut Butter Balls:

Ingredients:

- 2 cups puffed quinoa
- 1 cup peanut butter
- ½ cup agave nectar
- 2 tablespoons crushed roasted peanuts

Method:

1. Mix together in a large bowl peanut butter, agave and vanilla. If the mixture is too hard, then slightly warm it up until soft.
2. Add puffed quinoa and peanuts. Mix well and refrigerate for about 15-20 minutes.
3. Remove from the fridge, make small balls (lemon sized) from the mixture and refrigerate for a while before serving.

Chapter 7: Gluten free Appetizers' Recipes

Spiced Sweet Potato Wedges

Ingredients:

- 1 pound sweet potatoes, rinsed, chopped into wedges
- 1 teaspoon sumac
- 1 teaspoon chili flakes or to taste
- 1 teaspoon ground cumin
- 2 cloves garlic, minced
- 1 tablespoon fresh rosemary, chopped
- 1 tablespoon fresh thyme leaves, chopped
- Juice of half a lemon
- Zest of half a lemon, grated
- 1 ½ tablespoon olive oil

Method:

1. Smash together rosemary and thyme leaves, garlic, chili flakes, cumin, and sumac using a pestle and mortar.
2. Transfer into a bowl. Add oil, lemon juice, and lemon zest. Add sweet potatoes and toss well.
3. Place the wedges with its skin side down, in a single layer on a baking sheet. Bake in a preheated oven at 400 degree F until tender from inside and brown and crisp from outside.

Bruschetta with Warm Tomatoes

Ingredients:

- 8 slices gluten free French bread – refer chapter 1
- 5 cups grape or cherry tomatoes
- ¼ cup shallots, finely chopped
- 1/3 cup fresh basil, thinly sliced
- ½ teaspoon balsamic vinegar
- 4 teaspoons olive oil
- ¼ teaspoon freshly ground black pepper
- ½ teaspoon sea salt
- 1 clove garlic, halved
- 2 cloves garlic, minced
- Cooking spray

Method:

1. Add all the ingredients except bread, cooking spray and halved garlic to a bowl. Mix well and keep it aside for about an hour.
2. Place a nonstick skillet over medium heat. Spray with cooking spray. Add the tomato mixture and cook for about 10 minutes. Remove from heat and keep it aside.
3. Place a grill pan over medium high heat. Spray with cooking spray. Place the bread slices in batches and cook for a couple of minutes on each side until it is toasted.
4. Rub a side of toast with the halved garlic. Repeat with all the bread slices.

5. Spread tomato mixture over each of the toasts and serve immediately.

Beef Teriyaki Crisps with Wasabi Mayonnaise

Ingredients:

- 1 pound flank steak, trimmed of fat
- ½ cup low salt soy sauce (gluten free)
- ½ cup fresh orange juice
- ¼ cup honey
- ¼ cup mirin (sweet rice wine)
- 1 ½ tablespoons fresh ginger, peeled, grated
- 1 cup low fat mayonnaise
- 4 teaspoons wasabi paste
- 4 teaspoons rice wine vinegar
- 3 dozens gluten free rice crackers or multi grain crackers – refer chapter 6 or as many as required
- Fresh chives (optional), chopped
- Cooking spray

Method:

1. Mix together orange juice, soy sauce, mirin, honey, ginger and steak in a large zip lock bag. Seal the bag and place in the refrigerator to marinate for 12-24 hours. Turn the bag around occasionally.
2. Remove the steak from the zip lock bag and discard the marinade.
3. Place a grill pan over medium high heat. Spray with cooking spray. Add steak and grill until done. Flip

slides and grill the other side too. Remove steak from the pan and place on a plate.
4. When cool enough to handle, cut thin slices of the steak diagonally across the grain. Cut the slices into 2 inch pieces.
5. Mix together in a bowl, mayonnaise, wasabi paste, and vinegar.
6. Spread about ¾ teaspoon of the mayonnaise mixture over a cracker. Repeat with the remaining crackers. Divide the steak amongst the crackers and place over the crackers. Top again with mayonnaise mixture.
7. Garnish with chives and serve.

Marinated Shrimp on the Grill

Ingredients:

- 1 pound shrimp, peeled, deveined, tails attached
- ½ cup olive oil
- 2 cloves garlic, minced
- ½ tablespoon tomato paste
- 2 tablespoons fresh parsley, chopped
- 1 tablespoon hot pepper sauce
- Juice of half a lemon
- ½ teaspoon salt
- ½ teaspoon freshly ground black pepper
- 1 teaspoon dried oregano

Method:

1. Add olive oil, lemon juice, parsley, hot sauce, tomato paste, garlic, oregano, salt and pepper to a bowl. Retain a little and pour the rest over shrimp. Cover and marinate for 12-24 hours.
2. Preheat a grill to medium low heat. Meanwhile fix the shrimp onto skewers. Pierce it once near the head and once near the tail.
3. Oil the grill grate. Gill the shrimp for about 5 minutes per side or until it turns opaque. Use the retained marinade to baste it. Baste it frequently.

Lemon-Caper Parmesan Potato Salad Bites

Ingredients:

- 2 dozen small red potatoes, halved
- 1 cup light sour cream
- 4 teaspoons olive oil
- 4 tablespoons capers, drained, finely chopped
- 4 tablespoons butter, melted
- 4 tablespoons fresh chives, minced, divided
- 3 teaspoons lemon juice
- 1 teaspoon kosher salt
- 1 teaspoon freshly ground pepper
- 4 tablespoons parmesan, grated

Method:

1. Place potatoes in a bowl. Add oil and toss well.
2. Place the potatoes with its cut side down in a single layer on a baking sheet that is lined with parchment paper.
3. Bake in a preheated oven at 450 degree F for about 20 minutes. Turn the potatoes and bake for another 10 minutes.
4. Remove from the oven and set aside to cool.
5. Gently cut a circle in the cut part of the potatoes. Use a melon baller or a spoon and scoop out the pulp of the potatoes and keep it in a bowl. You are now left with a thin shell. Keep these shells aside.

6. Meanwhile, mix together the potato pulp, sour cream, half the chives, capers, lemon juice, salt, pepper, and butter. Mash well and fill the potato shells with this filling. Sprinkle cheese over it. Garnish with remaining chives.
7. Broil in an oven for a couple of minutes until the cheese is melted and light brown.

Chapter 8: Gluten free Soups Recipes

Moroccan Lentil Soup:

Ingredients:

- 1 onion, chopped
- 2 cloves garlic, minced
- ½ teaspoon fresh ginger, grated
- 4 cups water
- ½ cup red lentils
- ½ a 15 ounce can garbanzo beans, drained
- ½ a 19 ounce can cannellini beans
- ½ a 14.5 ounce can chopped tomatoes
- ½ cup carrots, chopped
- ¼ cup celery, chopped
- ¾ teaspoon ground cardamom
- ¼ teaspoon cayenne pepper
- ¼ teaspoon ground cumin
- ½ tablespoon olive oil

Method:

1. Place a large pot with olive oil over medium heat. Add onions, garlic and ginger. Sauté until the onions are translucent.
2. Add rest of the ingredients and bring to a boil.
3. Lower heat and simmer for about an hour or until the lentils are cooked.
4. Remove half the soup from the pot. Cool a little and blend with a stick blender.

5. Transfer the pureed soup back to the pot. Mix well, reheat and serve.

Pesto Chicken Soup:

Ingredients:

- 2 cups chicken stock
- 2 cups fresh spinach
- 1 cup cooked chicken, shredded
- 1 can (14 ounce) Great Northern or cannelloni beans, rinsed, drained
- 3 tablespoons pesto

Method:

1. Add all the ingredients except pesto to a saucepan and bring to a boil.
2. Lower heat and add pesto. Simmer for 2-3 minutes and serve hot.

Cream of Mushroom Soup:

Ingredients:

- 3 cups broth (vegetable or chicken)
- 1 1/3 cups milk
- 2/3 cup almond flour
- 1 cup mushrooms, chopped
- 1 tablespoon ground all spice

Method:

1. Place the broth, mushrooms and all spice in a pot. Place the pot over medium heat. Bring to a boil.
2. Mix together almond flour and milk and gently add to the pot stirring constantly.
3. Bring to a boil again and serve hot.

Turkey Tortilla Soup

Ingredients:

- 4 cups turkey, cut into ½ inch cubes
- 2 cups yellow onions, chopped
- 4 teaspoons olive oil
- 2 cans (4 ounce can) chopped green chilies
- 2 cans (15 ounce each) diced tomatoes with its juices
- 12 cups chicken or turkey broth
- 2 packages taco seasoning mix
- 2 cans (15 ounce) corn kernels, drained
- 1 cup crushed tortilla chips
- 2/3 cup fresh cilantro, chopped
- 1 cup Monterey Jack cheese, grated
- Salt to taste
- Pepper powder to taste

Method:

1. Place a large pot over medium heat. Add oil. When oil is heated, add onions and sauté until onions are translucent. Add chilies and taco seasoning. Mix well and simmer for a minute.
2. Add tomatoes and broth and bring to a boil.
3. Add corn and turkey. Mix well and simmer for about 30 minutes.

4. Garnish with tortilla chips, cheese and cilantro and serve.

Gazpacho

Ingredients:

- 4 pounds ripe tomatoes, washed, remove stems
- 2 cloves garlic, peeled
- 1 white onion, chopped
- 2 green bell peppers, deseeded, chopped
- 2 cucumbers (6-7 inches each), peeled, chopped
- ½ teaspoon cumin, powdered
- 6 tablespoons red wine vinegar
- 1 tablespoon salt or to taste
- 2 cups virgin olive oil
- 2 pieces French bread (each about 4 inches long) - refer chapter 1

Method:

1. Take a bowl of water. Soak the bread for a few seconds. Remove and squeeze with your hands any excess water from it.
2. Place all the ingredients in the food processor bowl. Blend on high speed until smooth and creamy.
3. Chill in the refrigerator. Lasts for a week.
4. Serve cold in bowls.

Chapter 9: Gluten free Main Course

Authentic Spanish Paella

Ingredients:

- 1 ½ cup bomba or calasprra rice or Arborio risotto
- 3 ½ cups chicken stock, hot
- ½ cup white wine
- 1 medium onion, diced
- 2 cloves garlic, minced
- 1 medium bell pepper, diced
- 8-10 flat green beans
- 2 plum tomatoes, diced
- 2 ounce tomato paste
- 8 large shrimp or prawns or clams or mussels or calamari
- 1 ½ pound rabbit meat or chicken legs
- 2 link chorizo sausages, sliced into 1 inch pieces
- 2 tablespoons fresh thyme, chopped
- ¼ cup fresh parsley, chopped
- 1 teaspoon paprika
- A pinch saffron threads
- 2 lemons, quartered

Method:

1. Slice the rabbit meat into small pieces. Season with salt.
2. Peel the shrimps with the tail on. Season with salt.

3. Place a large saucepan over high heat. Add olive oil and chorizo. Sauté until brown. Keep aside.
4. In the same pan add rabbit meat and sauté until brown. Remove and keep aside.
5. In the same saucepan add garlic, onion, and bell pepper. Sauté for a couple of minutes. Add tomatoes and sauté for a minute. Push all the vegetables to one side of the pan. On the other side, add tomato paste and caramelize it over high heat.
6. Now add the meat and mix together everything. Add paprika, thyme, and parsley.
7. Add rice and sauté for a couple of minutes. Add crushed saffron. Sauté until the rice is translucent.
8. Add chicken stock and wine. Keep the rice covered with broth. If it is less, add more broth. Lower heat and simmer. Stir a couple of times in the first 5-10 minutes. Add more broth if necessary to cover the rice.
9. After the first 10 minutes do not stir the rice. Keep adding broth until cooked if necessary so that the rice is submerged in the broth.
10. 8-10 minutes before the rice is fully done, place the shrimp on the top. Cook for 2-4 minutes. Turn the shrimps and cook the other side too for 2-4 minutes.
11. When the rice is almost al dente, remove from heat, and keep aside for 15-20 minutes. Now open the lid and serve hot garnished with lemon wedges.

Takikomi Gohan (Japanese Mixed Rice):

Ingredients:

- 3 cups white rice
- 4 ounce chicken thighs, skinless, boneless, cut into small pieces
- 4 carrots, chopped like matchsticks
- 4 button mushrooms, cut into pieces
- 2 cups stock
- ¼ cup sake
- 3 tablespoons gluten free soy sauce
- 1 teaspoon salt

Method:

1. Cook the rice as you usually do.
2. Sprinkle some sake on the chicken pieces and keep aside for 15 minutes.
3. Add stock, mushroom, chicken, and carrot to a pot. Place the pot on medium heat. Bring to a boil.
4. Add sugar and remaining sake. Simmer for a couple of minutes. Add soy sauce and simmer for 2 more minutes.
5. Remove all the solids from the pot and keep aside. Cool the remaining liquid.
6. Add the cooked rice into the remaining liquid. If you find it dry, then add some warm water. Stir well.

7. Add the solid ingredients back to the pot. Mix, cover, and cook for 10 minutes.
8. Serve in small bowls.

Tandoori Chicken:

Ingredients:

- 3 tablespoons Tandoori spice mix (Indian)
- 2 cups plain yogurt
- 2 pounds chicken, skinless, trimmed of fat, chopped
- 2 tablespoons ginger-garlic paste
- Salt to taste
- Chat masala (optional)
- 2 tablespoons lemon juice

Method:

1. Mix together in a bowl all the ingredients except chicken and chat masala.
2. Add the chicken. Mix well.
3. Cover and refrigerate for 4-5 hours.
4. Either grill it or roast in the oven at 400 degree F for about 30 minutes or until done. Tastes best when grilled.
5. Sprinkle chat masala and lemon juice Serve hot.

Chicken and Broccoli

Ingredients:

- 4 chicken breasts, skinless, boneless, cut into 1 inch pieces
- 2 bunches broccoli, cut into florets
- 1 cup green onions, sliced
- 4 tablespoons rice wine vinegar
- 6 tablespoons low sodium gluten free soy sauce
- 4 tablespoons honey
- 2 tablespoons cornstarch
- 1 teaspoon ground ginger
- 2 cloves garlic, minced
- 4 tablespoons olive oil
- 2 teaspoons sesame oil
- 2 teaspoons sesame seeds, toasted
- Salt to taste
- Pepper powder to taste

Method:

1. Place a large skillet over medium high heat. Add 2 tablespoons olive oil. When oil is heated, add chicken. Sprinkle salt and pepper over it. Cook until chicken is brown and is almost cooked.
2. Meanwhile add soy sauce, honey, rice wine vinegar, cornstarch, ginger, garlic, and sesame oil to a bowl and whisk well.

3. When chicken is brown, add broccoli to the same and stir. Cook until broccoli turns bright green in color. Add soy sauce mixture and stir constantly until the sauce thickens.
4. Remove from heat. Serve pork chops garnished with green onions and toasted sesame.

Shallow Poached Trout:

Ingredients:

- 10-12 slices lemon
- 4 leeks, halved, white and light green parts only
- 4 cups water
- 2 (8 ounce each) skin on trout fillet, boneless
- Salt and pepper to taste (optional)

Method:

1. Place a skillet over medium heat. Place the slices of lemon at the bottom.
2. Place the leeks over the lemons and add water.
3. Sprinkle salt and pepper over the trout. Gently place the fillets over the leeks.
4. Cover and simmer until the trout when pricked with a fork flakes easily.
5. Serve the trout hot along with the lemon, leeks, and liquid that are remaining in the pan.

Smoked haddock with lemon & dill lentils

Ingredients:

- 1 cup puy lentils
- 2 carrots, peeled, finely chopped
- 1 large onion, finely chopped
- 4 fillets smoked haddock fillets
- 2 sticks celery, finely chopped
- 4 cups vegetable stock
- 2 tablespoons half fat crème fraiche
- ¼ cup dill, chopped
- 1 cup baby spinach leaves
- Zest of a lemon
- Salt to taste

Method:

1. Add lentils, onion, carrot, celery and stock to a saucepan and bring to a boil.
2. Lower heat, stir, cover and simmer until lentils are cooked.
3. Add crème fraiche, half the dill, lemon zest, and salt to a bowl and mix well.
4. Place fish fillets in a microwavable dish. Sprinkle a little water and cover with cling wrap. Microwave on medium for 4 to 6 minutes or until the fish flakes easily when pierced with a fork.

5. Add spinach to the cooked lentils and cook for a couple of minutes until spinach wilts.
6. Add the crème fraiche mixture and stir.
7. Serve lentils in individual bowls. Place haddock over the lentils. Garnish with dill and serve.

Persian lamb Tagine

Ingredients

- 2 pounds lamb neck fillets, trimmed of fat, chopped into chunks
- 3 small onions, chopped into wedges
- 2 cloves garlic, finely chopped
- 3 tablespoons mild olive oil or any other vegetable oil
- ½ teaspoon ground turmeric
- 2 teaspoons ground coriander
- 2 teaspoons ground cumin
- ½ teaspoon chili powder
- A pinch saffron
- 1 stick cinnamon
- ¾ pound dried apricots
- ½ pound dates, pitted
- 1 preserved lemon, drained, chopped into wedges
- ¼ cup shelled pistachio
- 1 teaspoon rose water
- 2 tablespoons cornstarch
- Salt to taste
- Pepper powder to taste
- Cooked basmati rice to serve
- 2 tablespoons fresh cilantro, chopped

Method:

1. Season the lamb with salt and pepper.
2. Place a flameproof casserole dish over high heat. Brown the meat in 2 batches using a tablespoon of oil per batch. When done, transfer into a bowl.
3. Add remaining oil to the casserole dish. Lower heat to medium. Add onions and sauté until the onions are translucent.
4. Add garlic, cumin, coriander, chili and turmeric powders and sauté for a few seconds until fragrant. Add salt, pepper and browned lamb. Mix well and add 3 cups water, saffron, cinnamon stick and preserved lemon.
5. Let it begin to simmer. Stir in between a couple of times. Cover the casserole dish and place in a preheated oven at 350 degree F for about an hour.
6. Remove the dish from the oven and add apricots, dates and half the pistachios. Stir, cover and place it back in the oven.
7. Cook for about 30 minutes or until the lamb is cooked and soft.
8. Remove the dish from the oven and place over medium heat. Taste and adjust the seasoning if necessary. Mix together corn flour, rose water and 2 tablespoons cold water.
9. Add this mixture to the casserole dish stirring constantly until the sauce thickens.
10. Sprinkle remaining pistachio nuts over it. Garnish with cilantro and serve over cooked rice.

Apple Cinnamon Pork Chops

Ingredients:

- 6 ribs pork chops, bone in, about ¾ inch thick
- 4 ½ tablespoons butter, divided
- 2 medium onions, halved, thinly sliced
- 3 apples, cored, thinly sliced (peel if you desire)
- 3 teaspoons ground cinnamon
- 3 tablespoons packed brown sugar
- 1 cup apple cider vinegar
- ¼ teaspoon cayenne pepper
- Salt to taste
- Pepper powder to taste
- ½ cup heavy cream (optional)

Method:

1. Place pork chops in a bowl and season with salt and pepper. Keep it aside for a while.
2. Place a large skillet over medium high heat. Add 3 tablespoons butter. When butter melts, add pork chops and cook until brown on both the sides. Remove and place on a plate. Let it cool for about 3 minutes.
3. Place the skillet back on heat and add remaining butter. Add apples and onions and sauté until onions are translucent. Add brown sugar, cinnamon and cayenne pepper.

4. Add apple cider vinegar and cream and stir. Add pork chops and stir. Cook until done or internal temperature of pork shows 145 degree F on the thermometer.
5. Serve chops on a plate and spoon the apple mixture over it.

Beef Ragu:

Ingredients:

- ¾ pound beef, minced
- 3 tablespoons red pesto
- 2 teaspoons garlic infused butter
- 2 tablespoons fresh parsley, chopped
- Salt to taste

Method:

1. Place a nonstick pan over medium heat. Add 1-teaspoon garlic butter. When melted, add beef. Sauté until brown.
2. Lower heat. Add pesto and parsley. Sauté for a few minutes and transfer into a serving bowl.
3. Top with the remaining butter.
4. Serve with zucchini noodles (zoodles)

Teriyaki Tofu and Mushrooms

Ingredients:

- 1 package (14 ounces) firm tofu, sliced crosswise into 6 rectangles
- 1 ½ tablespoons fresh ginger, peeled, finely grated
- 2 tablespoons gluten free soy sauce or tamari or coconut aminos
- ½ tablespoon rice vinegar
- 1/2 tablespoon sugar
- 1 teaspoon cornstarch
- 1 tablespoon vegetable oil
- 2 cups fresh shiitake mushrooms, stemmed, caps sliced ¼ inch thick
- 3 cups, water cress, stemmed
- ½ cup water

Method:

1. Line a baking sheet with paper towels. Place the tofu slices on the paper towels in a single layer. Place paper towels over the tofu slices. Place a baking sheet over the tofu slices; Place something heavy on top of the 2nd baking sheet like a cast iron pan.
2. Let it remain like this for about 15 minutes. Most of the moisture should get absorbed by the paper towels.

3. To make the teriyaki sauce: Press the ginger through a fine strainer. Collect juice of the ginger and add to a bowl.
4. Add soy sauce, vinegar, sugar, cornstarch and water.
5. Place a nonstick pan over medium heat. Add ½ tablespoon oil. Add half the tofu. Cook until the bottom side is golden brown. Flip sides. Cook the other side to golden brown too. Remove onto a plate.
6. Repeat step 5 with the remaining tofu.
7. Add ½ tablespoon oil to the same pan. Add mushrooms and sauté until brown. Add teriyaki sauce and bring to a boil. Simmer until it thickens. If the sauce is thick, add some water to thin it.
8. Add the tofu back to the pan. Mix well to coat the tofu pieces with sauce.
9. Serve hot with watercress.

Chickpea Bajane

Ingredients:

- 2 cans (15 ounce each) chickpeas, unsalted, rinsed, drained
- 3 tablespoons extra virgin olive oil, divided
- 4 cups vegetable broth (gluten free)
- 2 cloves garlic, minced
- 2 cups quinoa, uncooked
- 2 cups water
- 4 cups leek, thinly sliced
- 4 tablespoons fresh thyme, chopped, divided
- 12 ounces fresh baby spinach
- 1 teaspoon salt, divided
- 8 cloves garlic, chopped
- 1 teaspoon fennel seeds
- 3 ½ cups carrots, peeled, sliced into ¼ inch thick slices
- 1 cup white wine
- 2 tablespoons fresh lemon juice
- ½ teaspoon freshly ground black pepper

Method:

1. Place a large saucepan over medium high heat. Add 1 and ½ tablespoons oil. When oil is heated, add minced garlic. Sauté until garlic is fragrant. Add 2

cups broth, quinoa, half the thyme and ½ teaspoon salt.
2. Bring to a boil. Lower heat, cover and simmer until quinoa is cooked and all the moisture is absorbed. Remove the saucepan from heat and fluff quinoa with a fork.
3. Place a large saucepan or Dutch oven over medium high heat. Add 2 teaspoons oil. When oil is heated, add leeks and chopped garlic to the pan. Sauté until onions are translucent.
4. Add remaining oil, fennel bulb, carrot and fennel seeds and sauté until vegetables are golden.
5. Add wine; cook until the wine almost dries up. Add remaining broth and thyme, and chickpeas. Heat thoroughly. Remove from heat and add juice, remaining salt, pepper and baby spinach.
6. Place about 2/3 cup of quinoa in individual serving bowls. Ladle about 1-½ cups chickpeas over quinoa. Garnish with remaining thyme and serve.

Soft Tacos with Green Chile–Cilantro Rice and Egg

Ingredients:

- 1 small onion, finely chopped
- 1 small tomato, chopped
- 2 tablespoons fresh cilantro, chopped
- 1 large egg
- 3 large egg whites
- 2 tablespoons fat free milk
- ½ tablespoon extra-virgin olive oil
- ½ a 4.5 ounce can chopped green chili, untrained
- 1 cup cooked brown rice
- ½ teaspoon ground cumin
- Salt to taste
- 4 gluten free corn tortillas
- Lime wedges to serve
- Cooking spray

Method:

1. Whisk together milk, egg and egg whites in a bowl and set aside.
2. Add onion, tomato, cilantro, oil, cumin, salt, rice, and green chilies to a bowl. Mix well, cover and keep it warm
3. Place a nonstick skillet over medium heat. Spray cooking spray all over the pan. Add egg mixture and

cook until it starts setting slightly. Now scramble the eggs such that you get bigger pieces but do not stir constantly.
4. Remove from heat.
5. Warm the tortillas according to the instructions given on the package. Divide the scrambled eggs among the tortillas and spread it. Divide the rice mixture and place over the scrambled eggs.
6. Fold over in the middle and serve with lime wedges.

Chapter 10: Gluten free Side Dishes

Zucchini Pasta

Ingredients:

- 3 medium zucchinis
- 9 tablespoons butter

Method:

1. Take a vegetable peeler and peel the zucchini into strips. Discard the seeds.
2. Place a nonstick pan over medium heat. Add butter.
3. When butter melts, add the zucchini strips. Sauté for 3-4 minutes stirring on and off.
4. Transfer on to a serving bowl and serve with any gluten free pasta sauce of your choice.

Zoodles (Zucchini noodles)

Ingredients:

- 1 medium zucchini
- 2 tablespoons butter

Method:

1. Make noodles of the zucchini using a spiralizer. If you do not own a spiralizer, then use a julienne peeler and peel the zucchini. Discard the seeds.
2. Place a nonstick pan over medium heat. Add butter.
3. When butter melts, add the zoodles. Sauté for 3-4 minutes stirring on and off.
4. Transfer on to a serving bowl and serve.

Bacon and Cheddar Mashed Potatoes

Ingredients:

- 1 1/4 pounds Yukon gold or baking potato, peeled, chopped
- 1/4 cup extra sharp cheddar cheese, shredded
- 1 apple wood smoked bacon slice, cooked, finely chopped
- 1/4 cup fat free milk
- 1/4 cup fat free sour cream
- 2 green onions, sliced
- 1/4 teaspoon salt or to taste
- Pepper powder to taste

Ingredients:

1. Place a saucepan filled with water over medium heat. Add potatoes and bring to a boil. Lower heat, simmer and cook until potatoes are soft. Drain and add it back to the saucepan.
2. Add milk and mash with a potato masher. Cook until thoroughly heated. Stir constantly as it is being heated.
3. Remove from heat; add cheese, sour cream, salt and pepper.
4. Garnish with green onions and bacon and serve.

Balsamic Roasted Asparagus

Ingredients:

- 2 pounds asparagus, remove the tough ends
- 2 tablespoons balsamic vinegar
- 2 tablespoons olive oil
- 1 teaspoon garlic, minced
- 1 teaspoon kosher salt or to taste
- 1/2 teaspoon freshly ground black pepper powder

Method:

1. Place the asparagus in a rimmed baking sheet. Sprinkle oil, salt, pepper, garlic and vinegar and toss well.
2. Bake in a preheated oven at 425 degree F for 10 minutes. Turn once in between.

Mexican Quinoa

Ingredients:

- 2 cups quinoa
- 1 large onion, chopped
- 2 jalapeno peppers, deseeded, chopped
- 2 tablespoons olive oil
- 2 cans (10 ounce each) diced tomatoes with green chili peppers and its juices
- 4 cups low sodium broth of your choice
- 2 envelopes taco seasoning mix
- 1/2 cup fresh cilantro, chopped
- Salt to taste

Method:

1. Place a large skillet over medium heat. Add oil. When oil is heated, add onions and sauté for a couple of minutes. Add quinoa and sauté for another 4 - 5 minutes.
2. Add garlic and jalapeno pepper and sauté for about a minute until garlic is fragrant.
3. Add tomatoes with green chilies, taco seasoning mix and broth. Bring to a boil.
4. Lower heat to medium low and simmer until all the broth has been absorbed by the quinoa.
5. Add cilantro, mix well and serve.

Braised Kale with Bacon and Cider

Ingredients:

- 4 bacon slices
- 2 1/2 cups onions, thinly sliced
- 2 pounds kale, chopped
- 3 cups Granny Smith apple, diced
- 1 teaspoon salt
- 1/2 teaspoon black pepper powder
- 2/3 cup apple cider vinegar

Method:

1. Place a skillet over medium heat. Add bacon and cook until it turns crisp. Remove the bacon with a slotted spoon and place on a plate lined with paper towels. When cool enough to handle, crumble the bacon.
2. Retain about a tablespoon of the bacon dripping and discard the rest.
3. Increase heat to medium high. Place the pan back on heat. Add onions and sauté until onions are translucent. Add kale and sauté until kale wilts. Stir frequently. Add apple cider vinegar, cover and cook for about 10 minutes.
4. Add apple, salt and pepper and cook until apples are soft. Stir occasionally.
5. Garnish with bacon and serve.

Chapter 11: Gluten free Desserts Recipes

Chocolate Pudding:

Ingredients:

- 4 cups fat-free milk or any milk of your choice
- 1 1/3 cup sugar
- 2/3 cup unsweetened cocoa
- 6 tablespoons cornstarch
- ¼ teaspoon salt
- 2 large eggs, beaten
- 8 ounce semisweet chocolate baking bar, chopped
- 2 teaspoons vanilla extract
- 2/3 cup thawed reduced-fat frozen whipped topping
- 2 tablespoons toasted almonds, slivered
- 2 tablespoons chocolate shavings

Method:

1. Place a heavy bottomed saucepan over medium heat. Add to it milk, sugar, cocoa, cornstarch and salt.
2. Whisk continuously until the mixture is hot.
3. Pour some of the milk into the egg. Mix well.

4. Pour the egg mixture into the saucepan gradually, stirring continuously until the mixture thickens. Remove from heat.
5. Add chocolate. Mix well until the chocolate melt. Add vanilla extract.
6. Transfer the contents in a serving glass dish.
7. Refrigerate for a couple of hours until the pudding is set and cooled well.
8. To serve, place into bowls and top with whipped topping, almonds and chocolate shavings.
9. For variation in taste: you can add a tablespoon of instant espresso powder.

Conclusion

With this, we have come to the end of this book. I sincerely hope you found the recipes interesting and easy to execute. All the recipes mentioned in this book are healthy and the ingredients easily available.

I hope your loved ones relish the recipes that you cook for them. Once again, thank you for choosing this book.

www.ingramcontent.com/pod-product-compliance
Lightning Source LLC
Chambersburg PA
CBHW071440070526
44578CB00001B/158